America Hernandez

Non-Hodgkin's Lymphoma: Nursing Process of Care

America Hernandez

Non-Hodgkin's Lymphoma: Nursing Process of Care

Patient undergoing chemotherapy and radiotherapy treatment

ScienciaScripts

Imprint

Any brand names and product names mentioned in this book are subject to trademark, brand or patent protection and are trademarks or registered trademarks of their respective holders. The use of brand names, product names, common names, trade names, product descriptions etc. even without a particular marking in this work is in no way to be construed to mean that such names may be regarded as unrestricted in respect of trademark and brand protection legislation and could thus be used by anyone.

Cover image: www.ingimage.com

This book is a translation from the original published under ISBN 978-620-2-16424-5.

Publisher:
Sciencia Scripts
is a trademark of
Dodo Books Indian Ocean Ltd. and OmniScriptum S.R.L publishing group

120 High Road, East Finchley, London, N2 9ED, United Kingdom
Str. Armeneasca 28/1, office 1, Chisinau MD-2012, Republic of Moldova, Europe
Printed at: see last page
ISBN: 978-620-6-51453-4

Table of Contents :

"APPLICATION OF A NURSING CARE PROCESS
TO A PATIENT WITH NON-HODGKIN'S LYMPHOMA UNDERGOING
CHEMOTHERAPY
TREATMENT
IN THE IMMUNOHEMATOLOGY WARD
OF THE CENTRAL MILITARY HOSPITAL".

SUMMARY

Non-Hodgkin's lymphoma is of great importance due to its high incidence and tendency to increase its frequency in recent years, statistics indicate that this trend will continue to rise, therefore it should be well known by the nursing staff. The application of a Nursing Care Process to a patient with non-Hodgkin's lymphoma, older than 18 years of age, with a hospital stay of more than seven days, indistinct sex, without relapse of the disease, without chronic degenerative diseases of infectious or metabolic type, without bone marrow transplant who wishes to participate in this project, will allow to verify whether or not benefits are obtained in the reduction of the symptoms of chemotherapy, establishing the appropriate interventions to prevent, help and achieve the patient's improvement.

Objective: To evaluate the benefits of the application of the Nursing Care Process on the side effects of chemotherapy in patients with non-Hodgkin's lymphoma in the Immunohematology ward.

Results: It is shown that nursing interventions produce a favorable evolution towards the improvement of the patient's needs according to the Virginia Henderson model, which were altered on admission. Considering the above information, a significant improvement in the objectives (NOC) of the PLACES can be observed, adding up to a positive result.

Chapter 1

I.INTRODUCTION

A. PROBLEM STATEMENT.

Based on the clinical file of the Hospital Central Militar during the last year (2015) 51 cases of non-Hodgkin's lymphoma were registered with a higher incidence in male patients over 70 years old, compared to the previous years 2013 with 31 cases and 2014 with 43 cases, it is remarkable the increase of this pathology, which requires that all nursing professionals must be constantly updated. Today the demands of the profession require knowledge of the Nursing Care Processes to provide competent, timely, effective and specialized care in order to provide care in a structured, logical and systematic manner.

The care of hematologic patients needs to introduce Nursing Care Processes that provide increasing expectations of improvement and thus indicate an adequate adjustment according to the patient's characteristics, adapting a management specific to non-Hodgkin's lymphoma.

What is the benefit that the Nursing Care Process will provide to decrease the side effects of chemotherapy for the patient with non-Hodgkin's lymphoma?

B. HYPOTHESIS.

The design of this proposed study and the objective of the study do not require a hypothesis or statistical testing of the hypothesis, but a working hypothesis was considered and is mentioned below:

Working hypothesis
The application of a Nursing Care Process in patients with non-Hodgkin's lymphoma helps to reduce the severity of the side effects of chemotherapy.

a. INDEPENDENT VARIABLE.

Application of a Nursing Care Process in the Immunohematology ward.

b. DEPENDENT VARIABLE.

Decrease the severity of chemotherapy side effects in patients with non-Hodgkin's lymphoma.

c. OBJECTIVES.

a. GENERAL.

To evaluate the benefits of the application of the Nursing Care Process on the side effects of chemotherapy in patients with non-Hodgkin's lymphoma in the Immunohematology ward.

b. SPECIFIC.

1. To have an organization of the activities to be carried out, managing time and resources needed.

2. To begin with the collection of data on the bedridden patient in the Immunohematology ward at the Hospital Central Militar by means of assessment instruments such as the Virginia Henderson nursing clinical history, prioritizing needs.

3. Specify the nursing interventions according to the needs that were diagnosed, thus obtaining nursing care plans.

4. To carry out the application of the Nursing Care Process to the bedridden patient in the Immunohematology ward of the Hospital Central Militar.

5. Record the evolution of the interventions by analyzing the results obtained with respect to the resolution of the patient's problems, modifying the interventions or data as necessary.

6. Write the analysis of results obtained after the application and evaluation of the process.

7. To demonstrate the benefits of having a nursing care process for a patient with non-Hodgkin's Lymphoma with chemotherapy treatment in the Immunohematology ward.

Chapter 2

II. RESEARCH PLAN

A. BACKGROUND.

Cancer is not a new disease. Egyptian papyri dating back to about 1600 B.C. already described it. It is believed that the Greek physician Hippocrates was the first person to use the word "carcinos" (crab) to describe cancer. When the first autopsy was performed by the Italian anatomist Giovanni Morgagni in 1761, the foundations were laid for the scientific study of cancer, also known as "oncology". In the 18th century, John Hunter was one of the first to suggest operating on a tumor. When the modern microscope was invented in the 19th century, the study of cancer began and the "modern pathological study of cancer" was born.

Non-Hodgkin's lymphoma is so named after Thomas Hodgkin is the first to describe abnormalities in the lymphatic system in 1832. Hodgkin believed that he had not been the first to discover the disease writing in his first article the following: "the morbid alterations of structure which I am about to describe are perhaps familiar to many practical morbid anatomists, as they are unlikely to have passed unnoticed during the course of cadaveric inspection", but that no one had documented and described in detail, the enlargement of the lymph nodes and spleen rejecting the possibility that the disease was caused by a primary inflammatory involvement. Unfortunately, most of the patients studied by Hodgkin reached an advanced stage of the disease and as he himself confessed: "there was nothing he could do for them as there were no therapeutic resources for the disease".

The cause of lymphoma was a matter of controversy for more than a hundred years, although its clinical and pathological manifestations were described, no one had been able to establish the origin of the disease. It was not until the 1960s when it was identified as a neoplastic disease.

The next step in chemotherapy was the discovery of vinca alkaloids, vincristine and vinblastine were used in clinical trials, in search of the perfect combination in 1963 the MOMP scheme was used (nitrogen mustard, vincristine, methotrexate and prednisone), the first study conducted with this scheme proved the expected improvement in remission.

B. CONCEPTUAL THEORETICAL FRAMEWORK.

a. Epistemology of care.

1. Domestic stage.

According to Marriner (2004) "this stage is called domestic because the woman is in charge of home care, which aims to maintain life in the face of adverse environmental conditions, through natural elements such as water, oils, skins, plants and hands, in order to maintain life through hygiene, food, clothing, and all basic care".

2. Vocational stage.

This stage is related to the birth of the Christian religion, for which the Christian society attributed health and illness to the designs of God and it was said that illness was a grace of the Almighty and that the one who suffers is God's chosen one. In this vocational stage the theoretical knowledge required by nurses was null and void with simple procedures, since they only required religious training. Nursing at this time is described as a religious activity of charity, submission and obedience (Marriner, 2004).

3. Etapatécnica.

It is the stage focused on the patient as the subject of the disease. Therefore, the main objective is the prevention of the disease. Scientific and technological development is applied to medical care, searching for the causes and treatments of the disease (Marriner, 2004).

Due to this technological complexity, it was necessary to have personnel to perform specific tasks such as diagnostic tests for curative purposes and drug administration; these people were called paramedical or auxiliary personnel, since they performed the tasks delegated to them by the physician (Marriner, 2004).

4. Professional stage.

Intervenes in a multidisciplinary team in order to effectively and autonomously attend to individual and collective health issues.

At the same time, research nurses emerge, who at a theoretical and philosophical level describe the differentiated performance of the profession, begin to use scientific work methods replacing the empirical, and the teachings are included in the university, where the stage of the professional nurse begins. (Marriner, 2004).

Dimensions of care.

i. Philosophical.

The philosophy of care possesses: universality, individuality, humility, alternate rhythms, patience, commitment, creativity, groundedness in knowledge, authentic presence and communication (Cavanagh, 2006).

ii. Anthropological.

It is defined as a scientific discipline in its interest in all human societies, past and present, covering a thematic field that includes aspects as diverse as language, social structure, belief systems and the political organization of different societies (Cavanagh, 2006).

iii. Ethical.

Nursing ethics studies the reasons for behaviors in the practice of the profession, the principles that regulate such behaviors, the motivations and values of professional practice, changes and transformations over time (Fry, 2010).

b. Nursing model and/or theory.

1. Theoretical generalities.

Virginia Henderson was born in 1897 in Kansas City and died in March 1996. It was in 1921 when she graduated as a nurse in the army school, and the following year she began her career as a teacher, which she completed with research, and which she did not abandon until her death. In 1922, Henderson began teaching nursing at a hospital in Virginia (Alligood, 2007).

In 1929 she worked as a faculty supervisor in the clinics of Strong Memorial Hospital in Rochester, New York. In 1953 she joined Vale University where she provided valuable input into nursing research. Henderson's model encompasses the terms Health-Care-Person-Environment from a holistic perspective (Alligood, 2007).

2. Meta paradigm of the model and/or theory.

Health: It is the quality of health rather than life itself; it is that margin of physical and mental vigor that allows a person to work at his or her maximum effectiveness and achieve a potentially higher level of life satisfaction (Alligood, 2007).

Care: It is aimed at making up for the deficits of autonomy of the subject in order to be able to act independently in the satisfaction of basic needs.

Environment: External factors that have a positive or negative effect on the person. The environment is dynamic in nature. It includes relationships with one's own family, as well as the responsibilities of the community to provide care (Alligood, 2007).

Person: as a being made up of biological, psychological, social and spiritual components that try to keep each other in balance. These components are indivisible and therefore the person is said to be an integral being.

Virginia Henderson stated that the nurse should not only assess the patient's needs, but also the conditions and pathological states that alter them, can modify the environment in cases where it is required and should identify the patient and family as a unit (Alligood, 2007).

3. Theoretical assumptions of the Virginia Henderson model.

It is the independence of the person in the satisfaction of the 14 fundamental needs:

i. First. Breathing normally.
ii. Second. Adequate eating and drinking.
iii. Third. Eliminate waste from the body.
iv. Fourth. Movement and maintenance of proper posture.
v. Fifth. Rest and sleep.
vi. Sixth. Select appropriate clothing.
vii. Seventh. Maintain body temperature.
viii. Eighth. Maintain body hygiene.
ix. Ninth. Avoidance of environmental hazards.
x. Tenth. Communicating with others, expressing emotions, needs, fears or opinions.

xi. Eleventh. To worship God, in accordance with religion.
xii. Twelfth. Work in a way that allows you to feel fulfilled.
xiii. Thirteenth. To participate in all forms of recreation and leisure.
xiv. Fourteenth. To study, discover or satisfy the curiosity that leads to a normal development of health. (Lanuza; et, al., 2008)

c. Nursing care process.

Describes Moran (2010) "process is a method of accomplishing something, usually involving a number of steps, that attempts to achieve a particular outcome. The nursing process is the application of scientific problem solving to nursing care. This process is used to identify the patient's problems, to systematically plan and carry out nursing care, and to evaluate the results obtained with this care".

1. Valuation.

The first phase of the nursing process is the assessment. Before the nurse can plan the care to be provided to the patient, she must identify and define the patient's problems. Consequently, this phase includes the collection of data about the patient's health status and ends with a nursing diagnosis, which is a report of the problems that afflict the patient (Alfaro, 2010).

One form of data collection is the nursing record which includes areas of assessment such as the patient's diagnosis and treatment, activities of daily living (grooming, eating, exercise, rest, relaxation and sleep habits), physical condition, psychological status, and a socioeconomic and cultural history, occupation, economic status, education, entertainment and religious customs. This written record of specific information about the patient provides the basis for assessing the patient's current and potential problems. It also serves as a basis for planning and delivering nursing care (Alfaro, 2010).

A survey of the patient's home and community are helpful for assessment, but may be difficult to perform. Other secondary sources for gathering information about the patient are current and past medical records, developmental records, computerized memos, nurse notes and visits, the kardex, and shift change reports.

This assessment allows the nurse to make a diagnosis, which is a report of the patient's problems, including their physical condition, limitations and how they adapt to the problem. This gives the nurse the opportunity to develop an individualized plan for the patient's care (Alfaro, 2010).

2. Diagnosis.

Nursing diagnoses are statements that establish problems that can be prevented, resolved or reduced by independent nursing action. There are 3 types of nursing diagnoses: actual, risk and health.

To make diagnoses we use the NANDA taxonomy and in PES format (problem, etiology and signs and symptoms) (Alfaro, 2010).

3. Planning.

The planning phase begins with the nursing diagnosis, which is elaborated through the collection and assessment of data involving nursing care (Alfaro, 2010).

In identifying the patient's problems, the nurse should set priorities, determining which are most urgent. Define immediate, intermediate and long-term objectives, or goals to strive for. The nurse and patient should define mutually acceptable goals. The patient and family should actively participate in care planning.

From the general objectives, the nurse can determine more specific objectives, which should be stated in terms of observable behavior. The nursing actions aimed at achieving the objectives, which can be classified as nursing interventions, management or treatment, should be explicitly stated in the nursing plan. The nursing care plan should be individualized so that it cannot be used for any other patient. It should include the patient's problems, goals, objectives and nursing interventions. With its elaboration, the planning phase is completed (Alfaro, 2010).

4. Execution.

If a plan is not put into action, it is not useful. Therefore, once the nursing intervention has been determined and the planning phase has been completed, execution of the plan begins. While executing the plan of care, the nurse continues to collect and assess data and plans, and evaluate care.

Execution is the actual delivery of nursing care. A plan contributes to providing comprehensive nursing care because it takes into account the patient's physical, psychological, emotional, spiritual, social and cultural, economic and rehabilitative needs. The care is personalized so that it is specific to each patient. The execution of the care plan also helps in the continuity and coordination of care. Without adequate planning and communication about the plan, the patient may experience discrepancies or duplication of care. The plan promotes the smooth flow of nursing care during all stages of the patient's illness, and coordinates the program for the rest of the health care team to perform diagnostic tests and various treatments in an appropriate sequence for the patient. Once the nursing actions have been completed, the implementation phase concludes.

5. Evaluation.

The final, but continuous phase of the nursing process is the evaluation or assessment of the outcome of the care provided. Was the care provided effectively? If so, why? If not, why not, how could care be improved? Assessment of patient progress is based on a comparison between the care that was successfully provided and the care that should have been provided by the nurse, health care team, patient, or family, as outlined in the goals of the plan of care. The assessment of patient progress indicates which problems were resolved, and which require reassessment and replanning (Alfaro, 2010).

Nursing care assessment is a feedback mechanism for judging quality, and is designed to improve nursing care by comparing current care to standards. Nursing assessment indicates whether nursing care is being provided adequately, and identifies areas requiring corrective action.

Although evaluation is considered the final phase of the nursing process, it does not end there. The evaluation only points out the problems that have been solved, those that need to be reassessed and planned, as well as those that have been carried out and reevaluated. The nursing process is a continuous cycle (Alfaro, 2010).

d. PATHOLOGY.

1. Concept.

According to Philip (2003), "Lymphomas are a heterogeneous group of B- or T-cell neoplasms that usually originate in the lymph nodes, lymphoid tissue associated with digestive tissue, skin or spleen. Any organ such as lung, thyroid, bones, brain, gonads, etc. can be affected. This is why non-Hodgkin's lymphoma groups together a heterogeneous group of malignant tumors; perhaps there is no other neoplastic disease with such a wide spectrum of clinical and biological behaviors".

The natural evolution of some of its variants is rapid and fatal. There are many types of lymphomas; although they share several characteristics, they vary in relation to the type of neoplastic cell involved, the growth pattern, the speed of cell division and tumor progression. B-cell lymphomas are more frequent than T-cell lymphomas (Gutierrez, 2014).

2. Epidemiology.

According to Gutiérrez (2014), "Non-Hodgkin's lymphomas account for approximately 4% of all malignant tumors and are responsible for 4% of cancer deaths. Although their incidence shows wide variations between countries, there is a global and progressive increase in the world year after year."

It has been reported in the literature that extranodal lymphomas constitute about 26% of all lymphomas. The most commonly affected sites are nasal cavity, oral cavity, pharynx, gastrointestinal tract, skin and central nervous system (Gutierrez, 2014).

The relative survival rate of patients with non-Hodgkin's lymphoma increased from 28% between 1950-54 to 53% between 1989-96, mainly in young adults and children. The estimated lifetime risk of developing non-Hodgkin's lymphoma is 2.08%. Non-Hodgkin's lymphoma is more common in men with incidence 19.2/100000, compared to 12.2/100000 in women. The average age at diagnosis is 65 years and the incidence increases in population groups between 80 and 84 years (Gutierrez,2014).

In Mexico, according to the last report of the Histopathological Registry of Neoplasms in Mexico in 2014, 5818 new cases of non-Hodgkin's lymphoma were diagnosed, representing 5.43% of all malignant neoplasms (Gutierrez, 2014).

3. Etiology.

Valencia (2012) writes that the cause or causes responsible for NHL are unknown. The following are a series of environmental and host factors that may contribute to their development.

i. Viruses: Some viruses can directly affect the DNA of lymphocytes, which helps transform them into cancer cells. Human herpesvirus type 8 (HHV8) can also infect lymphocytes, causing a rare type of lymphoma called primary effusion lymphoma.

ii. Autoimmune diseases, such as rheumatoid arthritis, systemic lupus erythematosus, have been associated with mucosa-associated lymphoid tissue-associated lymphomas (MALT lymphoma) of the stomach (Valencia et al, 2012).

iii. Body weight and diet: Being overweight and obese may increase your risk of non-Hodgkin's lymphoma. Other studies have suggested that high fat and meat intake may increase your risk.

iv. Ionizing radiation: Nuclear reactor accidents or patients who have received radiotherapy against some other cancers have a slightly increased risk of non-Hodgkin's lymphoma later in life (Valencia, et. al; 2012).

v. Chemical agents: Certain herbicides and insecticides may be associated with an increased risk (Valencia, et. al; 2012).

vi. Some genetic (inherited) syndromes can cause children to be born with a deficient immune system (Avila, 2001).

vii. Cytogenetics: oncogenes (chromosomal alterations and translocations).

viii. Age: In general, aging is a strong risk factor for lymphoma with the majority of cases occurring in people aged 60-69 years or older (Valencia, et al; 2012).

ix. Race, ethnicity, and geography: In the United States, whites are more likely to have non-Hodgkin's lymphoma compared to blacks or Asian-Americans (Valencia, et al.; 2012).

4. Pathological anatomy.

The lymphatic system is one of the main components of the immune system, which has the mission of defending the organism from external aggressions. The main cell of the lymphatic system is the lymphocyte, a white blood cell that helps fight infections. There are two main types of lymphocytes, B lymphocytes and T lymphocytes. Lymphocytes are found in the lymph nodes and other lymphatic tissues (such as the spleen or bone marrow) (Dermot, 2010).

The lymphatic system consists of the lymph, lymphatic vessels, lymph nodes, spleen, tonsils, thymus and bone marrow. Therefore, given the multiple locations of the lymphatic system, lymphomas can be located anywhere in the body (Juve, 2006).

1. Hematopoiesis.

Hematopoiesis is the process of formation of the cellular elements of the blood. It starts in the bone marrow in a small population of cells called pluripotent *stem cells* or stem cells (Juve,2006).

Hemopoietic organs.

(A) Bone marrow.

(B) Liver.

(C) Spleen.

(D) Timo.

5. Clinical picture:

Lymphadenopathies are, in general terms, the most common reason for consultation. The most frequent locations are the cervical, axillary and inguinal chains (Table 1.3). Lymphadenopathies are painless and of variable consistency. Other symptoms that may lead to diagnosis are compressive symptoms (superior vena cava syndrome, lymphedema, spinal compression, etc.), hepatomegaly, splenomegaly, bone pain, metabolic complications (Gutiérrez, 2014).

Table 1.2 (Fernández et. al., 2012).

Classification of Lymphomas
Clinically aggressive non-Hodgkin's lymphomas in WHO classification

Classification of Lymphomas
B-CELL NEOPLASIAS B-cell precursor neoplasms Leukemia/lymphoblastic lymphoma **Mature B-cell neoplasms** Mantle cell lymphoma Diffuse large cell lymphoma Mediastinal lymphoma Burkitt's lymphoma/leukemia Intravascular large B-cell lymphoma Cavity lymphoma
T AND NK CELL NEOPLASES Precursor T-cell neoplasms Lymphoblastic leukemia/lymphoblastic lymphoma Mature T-cell neoplasms Leukemic forms Adult T-lymphoma/leukemia **Cutaneous forms** Anaplastic large cell lymphoma **Extraganglionic forms** Intestinal T lymphoma with enteropathy Hepatosplenic T lymphoma Subcutaneous T-paniculitis NK lymphoma, nasal type Blast NK lymphoma **Ganglionic forms** Peripheral T lymphoma, all subtypes **Angioimmunoblastic** lymphoma Anaplastic lymphoma.

Table 1.3 (Gutiérrez, 2014)

PRESENTATION GROUP	SITE OR SYMPTOMS	CASES
GANGLIONAR	Tends to be contiguous; 25% have mediastinal mass; abdominal lymph node involvement with bulky mass is common.	55-75 %
EXTRANODAL	Main sites of presentation; gastrointestinal tract, Waldeyer's ring, skin.	20-40%
SYMPTOMATICS	Nonspecific symptoms of fatigue, nocturnal diaphoresis or weight loss.	5%

The most frequent anatomical areas affected are: gastrointestinal tract, central nervous system, lung, pleura, bones and skin. Adenomegaly may be accompanied by general symptoms such as anorexia, weight loss greater than 10% in 6 months, excessive night sweats and fever greater than 38°. NHL can appear at any age, but the increase is progressive from adolescence and especially from the age of 40 (Juve, 2006).

The following are adverse prognostic factors:

i.   Male sex.

ii. Age over 40 years old.

iii. B symptoms (anorexia, weight loss, nocturnal diaphoresis, temperature above
     38°).

iv. Advanced stage.

v.   Multiple extranodal involvement.

vi. Invasion of bone marrow, liver or central nervous system.

vii. Elevated LDH.

viii. Abdominal bulky disease.

ix. Failure of previous chemotherapy treatment.

The basis for scheduling an adequate treatment should take into account, in addition to
the histologic category and stage, the age, location and volume of the ganglion masses,
medical history and/or concomitant diseases and the general condition of the patient.
In less than 10% of patients there is fatigue, lack of appetite and weakness or intense
itching not localized in a specific area but generalized (Juve, 2006).

Other common symptoms include:
   i.   Inflammation of the lymph nodes.

   ii. Inflammation of the abdomen.

   iii. Feeling of fullness after eating only a small amount of food.

   iv. Chest pain or pressure.

   v.   Shortness of breath or cough.

   vi. Fatigue.

6. Complications.

    i. Myelosuppression is the decrease or annulment of the bone marrow function to produce blood cells, resulting in anemia (decrease in red blood cells and/or hemoglobin), thrombocytopenia (decrease in platelets) and leukopenia (decrease in white blood cells or leukocytes).

    ii. Stomatitis.

    iii. Hyperpigmentation.

    iv. Hepatotoxicity.

    v. Neurotoxicity.

    vi. Lethargy.

    vii. Transient elevation of transaminase and bilirubins.

    viii. Anaphylactic reactions.

    ix. Renal failure.

    x. Pancreatitis.

    xi. Carcinogenesis

    xii. Cardiotoxicity.

7. Diagnosis.

Definitive diagnosis can only be made by excisional biopsy of the pathologic lymph node or resection of the tumor tissue followed by a complete pathologic study, including immunology and histochemistry. Fine needle aspiration biopsy is not sufficient for the initial diagnosis of non-Hodgkin's lymphoma. The main pretreatment studies are described below (Table 1.4) (Feliu, 2001).

STUDIES PRIOR TO THE START OF TREATMENT.
ESSENTIAL STUDIES

- Complete medical history with record of growth velocity, symptoms present and functional status.
- Detailed physical examination with emphasis on lymphovascular areas and Waldeyer's ring. Lymph node and mass measurements
- Adequate excisional biopsy allowing morphological and immunohistochemical study of the specimen by an experienced pathologist.
- Laboratory tests:
  Complete blood count with erythrocyte sedimentation rate.
  Lactate dehydrogenase, calcium and uric acid.
  Renal and liver function tests.
  HIV.
- Radiological studies:
  Teleradiography of the thorax
  CT of the neck, thorax, abdomen and pelvis.
  Bone marrow aspirate and biopsy, including genetic and molecular analysis, if available.

OPTIONAL PROCEDURES DEPENDING ON THE CLINICAL PICTURE
- Endoscopy (e.g. gastric MALT).
- Planned radiographs, metastatic bone series or magnetic resonance imaging
- Positron emission tomography (PET).
- Cranial or spinal MRI (neurological symptomatology).
- Lymphography.
- Gammagraphies: bone, hepatosplenic, with gallium, etc.
- Lumbar puncture.
- Peripheral blood flow cytometry.
- Cerebrospinal fluid study in all patients at risk (infiltration or MO, centrofacial or testicular lymphoma, more than 2 extranodal sites.

Table 1.4. (Gutiérrez, 2014).

When making the diagnosis of non-Hodgkin's lymphoma, the stage according to Ann Arbor will be identified (Table 1.5).

ANN ARBOR CERTIFICATION SYSTEM.

CLINICAL STAGE	SITE OF AFFECTATION

I IE II IIE III IIIE IIIE IIIS IIISE IV	A single ganglionic region.
	Single organ or extranodal site.
	Two or more ganglionic regions on the same side of the diaphragm.
	An extranodal organ or site in addition to a stage I criterion.
Symptoms	Ganglionic regions on both sides of the diaphragm:
	+ an extranodal (localized) organ or site
	+ spleen
	+ spleen and a localized extranodal organ or site.
	One or more extranodal organs or sites with or without nodal involvement.
Bulky mass	A: absence of symptoms B.
	B: presence of at least one of the following:
	• Unexplained weight loss >10% in the 6 months prior to diagnosis.
	• Unexplained fever >38°.
	• Nocturnal diaphoresis.
	• Bulky: > 10 c.
	• Non voluminous: >10 cc.

Table 1.5 (Gutiérrez, 2014).

8. Treatment.

   i. Chemotherapy.

According to Hillman (2006) chemotherapy is the use of drugs to destroy cancer cells. It works by preventing cancer cells from growing and dividing into more cells. The drugs used in antineoplastic chemotherapy are called cytostatic or cytotoxic drugs.

Routes of administration of chemotherapy:
- (A) Intravenous chemotherapy.
- (B) Oral chemotherapy.
- (C) Intramuscular chemotherapy.
- (D) Chemotherapy in an artery or intra-arterially.
- (E) Chemotherapy in the peritoneum or abdomen.
- (F) Topical chemotherapy.

Anticancer drugs reach practically all the body's tissues, without differentiating between malignant and healthy cells. This causes a number of side effects in the patient, which generally disappear once the treatment is completed. The healthy cells that are most frequently damaged involve the cells of the bone marrow, digestive tract and hair follicle, resulting in the most common side effects of chemotherapy, which are:

i. Fluid accumulation or lymphedema.

ii. Skin conditions, dehydration, edema or fluid retention.

iii. Anemia.

iv. Hair loss or alopecia.

v. Changes in taste.

vi. Mental confusion or delirium.

vii. Diarrhea.

viii. Shortness of breath or dyspnea.

ix. Headaches.

x. Side effects on the nervous system.

xi. Constipation.

xii. Fatigue.

xiii. Hypercalcemia.

xiv. Infection.

xv. Fluid in the abdomen or ascites, fluid surrounding the lungs or malignant pleural effusion.

xvi. Mucositis

xvii. Peripheral neuropathy.

xviii. Neutrocytopenia.

xix. Intestinal obstruction or gastrointestinal obstruction.

xx. Weight loss, loss of appetite, nausea and vomiting.

xxi. Cognitive problems.

xxii. Coagulation problems

xxiii. Sleep problems: hypersomnia, drowsiness or insomnia.

xxiv. Dry mouth or xerostomia.

xxv. Symptoms of menopause in women.

xxvi. Infertility.

xxvi. Thrombocytopenia.

FIRST LINE TREATMENT			
SCHEME	PHARMACOTICS	SCHEME	PHARMACOTICS
CHOP	Cyclophosphamide Adriamycin Vincristine Prednisone (every 21 days)	**ProMACE**	Cyclophosphamide Adriamycin VP-16 Prednisone Methotrexate (+leucovorin)
R-CHOP	CHOP+ rituximab		
m-BACOD	Methotrexate (+Leucovorin) Bleomycin Adriamycin Cyclophosphamide Vincristine Dexamethasone (every 21 days)	**MOPP**	Mechlorethamine Vincristine Procarbazine Prednisone
CytaBOM	Adriamycin VP-16 Prednisone Cytarabine Bleomycin Vincristine Methotrexate (+leucovorin)	**MACOP**	Cyclophosphamide Adriamycin Vincristine Methotrexate Bleomycin Prednisone
SECOND-LINE TREATMENT			
ICE:	Ifosfamide Carboplatin Etoposide	**GVD, Gem-Ox, or GDP:**	Gemcitabine Vinorelbine Doxorubicin Gemcitabine Oxaliplatin Gemcitabine Dexamethasone Cisplatin.
ESHAP or DHAP:	Etoposide, Methylprenisolone Cytarabine Cisplatin Dexamethasone	**Brentuximab vedotin (Adcetris**	Brentuximab-Vedotin

Table 2.1 Chemotherapy treatment scheme (Fernandez, 2005).

ii. Radiotherapy.

It consists of the use of high-energy radiation to kill cancer cells. Radiation treatment can be performed alone or with chemotherapy. Radiation therapy is a local treatment that affects only the cancer cells in the treated area. There is no radioactivity left in the body when the treatment is completed. Radio-immunotherapy is a combination of immune agents (such as rituximab) with radioactive isotopes, and offers some benefits by treating tumors locally at the molecular level. Sometimes patients receive chemotherapy or radiation therapy to kill undetected cancer cells that may be present in the central nervous system (CNS). In this treatment, called central nervous system prophylaxis, the doctor injects anticancer drugs directly into the cerebrospinal fluid (Fernandez, 2005).

iii. Bone marrow transplant.

It may also be a treatment option, especially in patients whose non-Hodgkin's lymphoma has relapsed (come back). Bone marrow transplantation provides the patient with healthy shock cells (very immature cells that produce blood cells) to replace cells damaged or destroyed by high doses of chemotherapy or radiation therapy. Healthy bone marrow can come from a donor, or also from the patient's own bone marrow from which it was previously obtained, treated to destroy cancer cells, stored, and returned to the patient after high-dose treatment. Until the transplanted bone marrow begins to produce enough white blood cells, patients must be carefully protected from infection to avoid infection. They usually stay in the hospital for several weeks and then in environments with a low probability of contagion (isolation measures). (Fernandez, 2005).

C. METHODOLOGICAL.

a. Study approach

This is an instrumental, holistic, experimental or interventional, prospective, single case study; longitudinal (before and after pre- and post-intervention).

Mixed. In the first stage, one part of the study is approached quantitatively and the other qualitatively, with a predominance of the quantitative part.

b. Type of study: Intervention.

c. Population.

Male or female subjects with non-Hodgkin's lymphoma who come to the immunohematology department, which may present certain characteristics susceptible to be studied.

d. Sample.

Patient with non-Hodgkin's lymphoma who meets the inclusion criteria.

e. Location.

Central Military Hospital, Immunohematology Department.

f. Time:

The protocol was initiated in September 2015, with the time of search and recruitment of the case for the study during the months of January-February 2015, a total of 10 interviews were conducted, which recruited or captured a patient who met all the criteria for inclusion in the study and the conclusions were made during the months of April-May 2016.

g. Criteria.

   1. Inclusion:
     i. Patient with non-Hodgkin's lymphoma undergoing chemotherapy (radiotherapy as secondary treatment).
     ii. Age >18 years old.
     iii. Sex indistinct.
     iv. Hospital stay of more than 7 days.

   2. Exclusion:
     i. With chronic degenerative diseases of infectious and metabolic type.
     ii. Relapse of the disease.
     iii. Hospital stay of less than 3 days.
     iv. With bone marrow transplant.
     v. Do not wish to participate in this process.

h. Ethical considerations.

All the proposed procedures are in accordance with ethical standards, as stipulated in NOM-012-SSA3-2012, the Regulations of the General Health Law on Health Research, title two, chapter I, article 17, section I, and with the Helsinki Declaration of 1975, amended in 1989, and current international codes and standards of good clinical research practice. Patient confidentiality was guaranteed and the information obtained will be entirely for the purpose of analysis and, if necessary, statistical procedure for research purposes; the protocol was approved by an ethics and research committee. It is considered a research without risk.

i. Techniques, instruments and procedures for data collection.

**BASIC NEEDS" MODEL
BY VIRGINIA HENDERSON
CLINICAL NURSING ASSESSMENT**

GENERAL DATA		
DATE: **15/02/2016** TIME: **09:10 A.M.**		FR: **18**
NAME: **E.M.R.**		FC: **85**
SEX: **MALE.** AGE: **21 YEARS**		TA: **110/80**
ADDRESS: **SAN ISIDRO, HUAYAPA, MIXE, OAXaCA.**		TEMP: **36**
DIAGNOSIS: **NON-HODGKIN'S LYMPHOMA.**		WEIGHT: **81 KG.** HEIGHT: **1.71 MTS**
REASON FOR ADMISSION: **PATIENT UNDER SURVEILLANCE FOR CHEMOTHERAPY.**		OCCUPATION: **MUSICIAN.**
		MARITAL STATUS: **SINGLE.**

1. BASIC NEED FOR OXYGENATION					
RESPIRATORY RATE: 18	**CHARACTERISTICS OF LUNG SOUNDS**	NORMAL X	ALTERATIONS	**TOS**	YES
		SIBILANTS	ASSOCIATED PAIN BREATHING		
		ESTERNOTES	NASAL ALETEUS		NO X
		PROLONGED	INTERCOSTAL PULL		
TOS SINO X	COUGH TYPE: N/A	DYSNEA	DOES NOT PRESENT X		

	PAROXISTICS		OCCASIONALLY	
	WITH SPUTO		HABITUAL	
	HEMOPTISIS		EACH PHYSICAL ACTIVITY	
	SECA		WHEN SLEEPING	
CYANOSIS	NO	**CHARACTERISTICS OF RESPIRATION:**	RHYTHMICS X	**THORACIC DEFORMITIES**	NO X
	CENTRAL		BRADIPNEA		PIGEON THORAX
	PERIPHERAL		TAQUIPNEA		FUNNEL THORAX
	ENTEROGENEA		OTHER		OTHERS:
SMOKER: SINO X ACTIVE LIABILITIES N/A	**CIGARETTES PER DAY:**	N/A	**AGE AT WHICH HE STARTED SMOKING:**	N/A

HISTORY OF CARDIORESPIRATORY DISEASES: ASTHMA   TACHYCARDIAPRECORDIAL PAIN

2. BASIC NUTRITIONAL AND HYDRATION NEEDS

No. OF MEALS PER DAY: 3				
	FOOD ALLERGIES: DENIED	**APPETITE IN THE HOSPITAL**	NORMAL	**TYPE OF DIET:** NORMAL 2000 KCAL.
			INCREASED	**AMOUNT OF LIQUIDS INGESTED:**
			DECREASED X	1 AND A HALF LITERS.
DIFFICULTY IN SWALLOWING:	NONE X	NASOGASTRIC TUBE		**CONTRAINDICATED FOODS:** RAW FOODS.
	TO SWALLOW SOLIDS	DOES NOT TOLERATE DIET		
	TO SWALLOW LIQUIDS	REFLUX		**MEAL TIMES PER DAY:** 07:00, 13:00 AND 18:00 HRS.
	NAUSEA	OTHERS: DISGUST FOR SMELL AND TASTE OF FOOD.		**SUPPLEMENTS:** NONE
SIGNS OF MALNUTRITION	NONE	**COMPLETE DENTURE**	YES X	**ALCOHOL CONSUMPTION**	YES
		FALL OF HAIR X			
	PALE	DRY HAIR	NO		NO X

DRY AND FLAKY SKIN X	MUSCULAR HYPOTONIA	CARIES	ULCERAS ORAL X	FREQUENCY: N/A	
		CUM INFLAMMATION		PAIN	PIROSIS
MUSCLE SPASMS	EDEMA	DIGESTIVE DISORDERS:		ACIDITY X	EMESIS X
				FLATULENCIES	OTHER
WEIGHT LOSS:	YES	NOX	BMI: 27.7	**WEIGHT: 81 KG.**	**HEIGHT: 1.71 MTS.**

LIKES OR DISLIKES: DISLIKES TO CHAYOTE, TUNA AND BOILED CARROT.

OBSERVATIONS: DIMINISHED SENSE OF TASTE.

3. BASIC NEED FOR DISPOSAL

NUMBER OF EVACUATIONS: 1 TIME PER DAY QUANTITY: NORMAL	CHARACTERISTICS:				NONE	AID:
	YELLOW: X		STRENGTH		STRENGTH	ENEMAS
		DIARRHEA				
		PASTOSA X	HEMORROIDS	ALTERATIONS:	HEMORROIDS	FOOD
	GREEN:					
	COFFEE:	LIQUID	INCONTINENCE		INCONTINENCE	MEDICATIONS
	BLACK:	SEMILIQUID	OTHERS:		OTHERS:	LIQUIDS

REMARKS:	AUTONOMY TO GO TO THE BATHROOM.

URINARIA

MICCIONES AL DAY: 4 TO 6 TIMES PER DAY	CHARACTERISTICS		ALTERATIONS	NONE X	HEMATURIA	ENEURESIS
	CLARA X YELLOW	NO ODOR		TENESMO	ANURIA	OTHERS:
		WITH THE SMELL OF MEDICINE		DISURIA	ESCOZOR	
	PARDA			NICTURIA	POLYACHIURIA	
	CONCENTRATED	OTHER				

AXIAL DIMENSIONS	INTERMITTENT PROBING		COVER	NONE
	PERMANENT PROBING		OTHER	
GENITALS			**REMARKS:** WHEN RECEIVING MORE CONCENTRATED AND ODOROUS URINE TREATMENT.	
ALTERATIONS:		**TYPE OF ALTERATION:**		
YES	NO X	ERUPTIONS	SECRETIONS	IRRITATION

4. MOVE AND MAINTAIN GOOD POSTURE

					CANE	**ALTERATIONS**	
MOVEMENTS	AUTONOMOUS		**LIMITATIONS IN AMBULATION.**				
	ASSISTED WALKING OR SITTING				MULETAS	FATIGUE	DECUBITUS ULCERS:
	RELATIVE IN BED ONLY GOES TO THE BATHROOM X				WALKER	WEAKNESS	
					WHEELCHAIR	JOINT STIFFNESS: OCCASIONAL	PARESTHESIA
	ABSOLUTE REST				NONE X		PAIN
POSITION	DC. DORSAL X	DC. VENTRAL	DC. RIGHT SIDE.	DC. LEFT SIDE X		SEMIFOWLER	FOWLER
HYGIENIC MEASURES WHEN MOVING		YES	NO X	**MAINTAINS** GOOD POSTURE	YES X	NO	
PHYSICAL EXERCISE		YES	NO X	**TYPE OF EXERCISE:** N/A SIVE			ACTIVOPAS

5. BASIC NEED FOR REST AND SLEEP

	ALTERATIONS			USE OF VOLTAGE REDUCERS: SINO X	PHARMACOTICS
HOURS OF SLEEP PER DAY: 14 HOURS	INSOMNIA	HYPERSOMNIA	NIGHTMARES		HERBOLARIA
	SOMNOLENCE X	NIGHT SWEAT	ANXIETY		MASSAGE
	FEAR	DIFFICULTY IN BREATHE	PAIN		MUSIC

REMARKS:				READING

6. BASIC NEED TO WEAR APPROPRIATE CLOTHING				
ACCEPTS HOSPITAL LINEN	SI **X**	NO	**WEAR SPECIAL CLOTHING**	YES	NO **X**
DIFFICULTY DRESSING	YES	NO **X**	**ALIÑO**	ADEQUATE **X**	INADEQUATE
FINANCIAL RESOURCES TO WEAR CLEAN CLOTHES:				YES	NO

7'. BASIC NEED FOR THERMOREGULATION					
SITE OF TOMA:	AXILAR X	VAGINAL	**ALTERATIONS:**		**PROTECTION AGAINST TEMPERATURE CHANGES**	
	RECTAL	INGUINAL	HYPERTHERMIA	COLD SKIN X	**YES** X	NO
	BUCAL	REGISTRATION: **T: 36° C**	HYPOTHERMIA	SCALOSPHROSPHROS		
			NIGHT SWEATS X			
OBSERVATIONS: NIGHT SWEATS ARE OCCASIONAL.					

8. BASIC NEED FOR SKIN HYGIENE AND PROTECTION						
BATH	**HAIR WASHING**	YES X	SELF-EMPLOYED X	**FREQUENCY:** DIARIO		HEMATOMAS
AUTONOMOUS X		NO	ASSISTED			CICATRIES
ASSISTED	**ORAL HYGIENE**	YES **X**	SELF-EMPLOYED X	**FREQUENCY:** DIARIO	**SKIN ALTERATIONS:**	DEHYDRATION CUTANEOUS **X**
OF SPONGE		NO	ASSISTED			
HAND WASHING		YES X	NO			DECLAMATION X
ALTERATIONS OF THE ORAL MUCOSA:	MUCOSITIS	STOMATITIS	GINGIVORRAGIA	ODONTALGIA	GINGIVITIS	
REMARKS:	DERMATITIS IN THE INGUINAL AREA DUE TO RADIOTHERAPY SESSIONS.					

9. NEED FOR SAFETY AND SECURITY				
STATE OF ALERTNESS:	ALERT X	**DRUG ALLERGY:** DENIED	**INSULATION:**	YES	**TYPE OF INSULATION:** PROTECTIVE
	ORIENTED X			NO	

	AWARE X		RISK OF FALLING:	YES X	SECURITY MEASURES:	MEDICATION
	UNCONSCIOUS			NO		BARANDALES
	STUPOR		SURVEILLANCE	SI X		FASTENERS
	COMA			NO		OTHERS:

HABITS THAT AFFECT PERSONAL SAFETY:	CHARACTERISTICS THAT CONSTITUTE A HAZARD IN YOUR HOME:	HEALTH RISKS:
DRINKS COFFEE, SUGARY SOFT DRINKS AND EATS FATTY OR STREET FOODS AT HOME.	SHE LIVES ON THE THIRD FLOOR SO SHE HAS TO CLIMB STAIRS, OCCASIONALLY THERE IS NO WATER SUPPLY IN HER HOME.	RISK OF INFECTION BY NUETROPENIA, PERCEPTIBLE TO ALLERGIES.

10. BASIC NEED FOR COMMUNICATION AND SEXUALITY

LANGUAGE: ENGLISH DIALECT: MIXE	ALTERATIONS				ADDITMENTS	APPARATUS AUDITORY: **NO**
	AFASIA	SIGN COMMUNICATION		MENTAL ILLNESS		
	DISERTRY	MUDEZ	MUTISM			
	DEAFNESS	TARTAMUDEZ	NINGUNAX	INSULATION		LENSES: **NO**

DO YOU FIND IT HARD TO EXPRESS YOUR FEELINGS ABOUT YOUR CONDITION? WHY? YES, BECAUSE YOU DON'T LIKE YOUR FAMILY TO SUFFER.	DO YOU ASK FOR HELP WHEN YOU NEED IT: NO, IT EXPRESSES TO GET STRONG

THE RELATIONSHIP IS YOUR FAMILY IS:	GOOD **X**	MALA	REGULAR

ONSET OF SEXUAL RELATIONS: 18 YEARS OLD	USES A CONTRACEPTIVE METHOD: CONDOMS.

YOUR CURRENT SEXUAL ACTIVITY HAS:	INCREASED	NORMAL	DECREASED **X**

FEELINGS OR SITUATIONS THAT AFFECT THEIR SEXUALITY:	FEAR FOR NOT KNOWING THE EFFECT OF THE DISEASE ON HER FERTILITY AND FOR NOT KNOWING IF SHE WILL BE ABLE TO HAVE CHILDREN IN THE FUTURE.

11. BASIC NEED FOR BELIEFS AND VALUES

RELIGION:		IS YOUR RELIGION IMPORTANT TO YOU?		DO YOU HAVE CONFLICTS BETWEEN YOUR BELIEFS AND HEALTH ISSUES?
CATHOLIC X	CHRISTIAN			NONE
JEHOVAH'S WITNESS	MORMONS	YES X	NO	

OTHER:	SPECIAL (RELIGIOUS) REQUESTS: IF AT ANY TIME YOU WOULD LIKE TO GO TO CONFESSION.

12. BASIC NEED FOR WORK AND SELF-FULFILLMENT

PREVIOUS EMPLOYMENT: MUSICIAN	ANXIETY ABOUT EMPLOYMENT DUE TO ILLNESS? YES NOW WHO IS NOT USED TO BEING OUT OF WORK
CURRENT EMPLOYMENT: NOT WORKING	ANGUISH BECAUSE OF ECONOMIC ISSUES? YES, BECAUSE HIS FAMILY DEPENDS ON HIM.
ACTIVITIES HE WOULD LIKE TO PURSUE: PLAYING THE TROMBONE AND BARITONE	

13. BASIC NEED FOR SELF-FULFILLMENT.

ACTIVITIES HE WOULD LIKE TO DO: PLAYING MUSICAL INSTRUMENTS.	FAVORITE ACTIVITIES			FACTORS THAT MAKE IT DIFFICULT FOR THEM TO BE DISTRACTED WHILE HOSPITALIZED:	PAIN
	READ	SPORTS	PLATICAR X		WEAKNESS X
	LISTEN MUSIC X	WALK	SURFING THE INTERNET X		ANGUSTIA X
REMARKS:		PLAY CARDS	TRAVEL		DEPRESSION
	CHESS	SLEEP X	DANCE		SOLEDAD

14. BASIC LEARNING NEEDS.

ACADEMIC LEVEL		ARE YOU INTERESTED IN LEARNING ABOUT YOUR DISEASE?			
ANALPHABET	HIGH SCHOOL X	YES X	NO		
PRIMARY	UNIVERSITY	HOW WOULD YOU RATE YOUR NURSING KNOWLEDGE?			
SECONDARY	MAESTRIA	NULO	POCO X	REGULAR	SUFFICIENT
OBSERVATIONS: VERBALLY EXPRESSES THAT SHE WOULD LIKE TO KNOW MORE ABOUT HER ILLNESS.					

SECRETARIAT OF NATIONAL DEFENSE.

DIR. GRAL. EDUC. MIL. AND RECT. OF THE U.D.E.F.A.
ESC. MIL. DE ENFRAS. SEC. INV. AND DOC. MIL.

REQUIREMENTS PRIORITIZATION

Need	Observed data

Need	Objective data / Subjective data
Oxygenation.	Respiratory rate 16 rpm, oxygen saturation 96%. Parched nostrils.
Nutrition and Hydration.	Admissions of 300gr and below, anorexia are recorded. He reports lack of appetite and nausea before, during and after treatment.
Elimination.	Records on nursing chart daily evacuation and unchanged. He refers to changes in the characteristics of urine during treatment, expressing that it is more concentrated and smells like medicine, urinating 4 to 6 times a day.
Moving and maintaining good posture.	Absolute rest due to myelosuppression and medical indication. Maintains good posture and balance when walking, observed when getting up to go to the bathroom.
Rest and Sleep.	She records 12 hours of sleep, refers decreased exercise tolerance. Occasional night sweats are reported. Somnolence is observed during the day.
Use of Appropriate Clothing.	Proper dressing. Use hospital clothing.
Thermoregulation.	Currently normo-thermal, but temperature is recorded in previous days without data of infection, it is related to side effects of chemotherapy.
Skin Hygiene and Protection.	Dermatitis in the groin area due to radiation sessions. Dehydrated and scaly skin. Thick and dry skin, skin lesion in the inguinal area, no pain, only itching. Oral mucositis in lower lip on the right side which causes pain and discomfort when eating. Daily bathing and daily teeth brushing.
Security	She is kept under surveillance due to myelosuppression and protective isolation is maintained as she is predisposed to infections. Your family and health care team use mouth covers and perform hand washing before visiting you.
Communication and Sexuality.	He is cooperative but has difficulty expressing his feelings. At the interview he expresses to be strong in front of his family. Diminished libido. Concern about his fertility.
Living according to Values and Beliefs.	Catholic. Belief in a God and feels faith. His beliefs do not interfere with his treatment.
Work and fulfillment.	He feels discomfort for not carrying out his daily life. He says that he stopped working 1 year and 1 month ago because of his illness and feels unproductive.
Participate in recreational activities.	Decreased social interaction due to illness. Expresses that he would like to return to his musical group.
Learning.	Lack of information about his pathology, so he expresses doubts about his disease and your treatment. The accompanying family member expresses doubts about the role of caregiver that corresponds to him/her.
Need	
	Objective data Subjective data

Nutrition and Hydration.	Intake lower than metabolic needs, abundant nausea and poor appetite. Alteration in the sense of taste, paleness of mucous membranes is observed.
Security	Decreased ability to protect oneself from internal or external threats such as illness or injury. No signs or symptoms of localized systemic infection were observed, but due to the diagnosis and being in the surveillance stage due to myelosuppression, the patient is kept under observation.
Learning.	Patient and family show deficiencies in the knowledge of the disease, for which a set of actions should be prepared with the aim of learning
Skin Hygiene and Protection.	Alteration of the dermis due to radiotherapy treatment. Scaly and dry skin texture. Oral mucositis due to chemotherapy treatment. Skin care planning.
Rest and Sleep.	Drowsiness due to which the quantity and quality of sleep is disturbed.
Need to Communicate.	Decreased ability to convey feelings and ideas. Cooperative but with low interaction with family members.
Sexuality and Reproduction.	Ineffective sexual pattern. Expresses doubts about fertility.
Participate in recreational activities.	Low tolerance to activity. Avoids strenuous activities. Does not engage in any recreational activity in the hospital or at home.

NURSING CARE PLAN						
NURSING DIAGNOSIS (NANDA)	*CLASSIFICATION OF NURSING OUTCOMES (NOC)*					
	RESULT	INDICATORS	MEASURING SCALE	TARGET SCORE		
				KEEP	INCREASE	
DOMAIN: 2 NUTRITION **CLASS:** 1 INGESTION. **CODE:** 00002 **Label (problem) (P)** Nutritional imbalance: intake below requirements. **Related factors (causes) (e)** Biological factors. **Defining characteristics (signs and symptoms)** It expresses alteration in the sense of taste, inflammation in the oral cavity, nausea and lack of appetite.	**DOMAIN:** V PERCEIVED HEALTH **CLASS:**V SITOMATOLOGY **CODE:** 2106 **EXPECTED RESULT:** NAUSEA AND VOMITING: ADVERSE EFFECTS	- DECREASED FOOD INTAKE. - DENIAL IN THE INGESTION OF FOOD.	1. SERIOUS. 2. SUSTANTIAL 3. MODERATE 4. LEVE 5. NONE	KEEP 2 KEEP 3	AUMENTA 4 AUMENTA 4	

INTERVENTIONS (NIC)	INTERVENTIONS(NIC)
NUTRITION MANAGEMENT ACTIVITIES: 1. Ask the patient if he/she has any food allergies. 2. Determine, in collaboration with the dietitian, the number of calories and type of nutrients needed to meet dietary requirements. 3. Provide light meals. 4. Perform meal selection.	**MANAGEMENT OF NAUSEA ACTIVITIES:** 1. Observe learning strategies to control nausea. 2. Perform complete assessment of nausea, including frequency, duration, intensity and triggers. 3. Evaluate past experiences with nausea. 4. Ask the patient about the foods he/she likes and dislikes the most. 5. Ensure that effective antiemetics have been administered to prevent nausea.
5. Ensure that the diet includes foods rich in fiber to avoid constipation. 6. Provide the patient with nutritious, high-calorie, high-protein foods and beverages that can be easily consumed, if appropriate. 7. Provide adequate information about nutritional needs and how to meet them.	6. Control environmental factors that may evoke nausea (visual estimation, bad smells, etc.). 7. Reduce or eliminate personal factors that trigger or increase nausea (anxiety, fear, fatigue, etc). 8. Teach the use of non-pharmacological techniques: relaxation, simple imagination, music therapy and distraction. 9. Encourage adequate rest and sleep to facilitate relief of nausea. 10. Administer cold food, clear, odorless and colorless liquids, as appropriate. 11. Weigh the patient regularly. 12. Recording of income.

BIBLIOGRAPHY: NANDA International 2012-2014, Moorhead, s. (2014) Nursing Outcomes Classification (NOC), Barcelona, Spain.
Elsevier., Bulechek, g. (2014) Nursing Interventions Classification (NIC), Barcelona, Spain. Elsevier.

DIR. GRAL. EDUC. MIL. EDUC
RECTOR OF THE U.D.E.F.A.

. MIL. OF ENFRAS.
SEC. INV. AND DOC. MIL.

NURSING CARE PLAN

NURSING DIAGNOSIS (NANDA)	*CLASSIFICATION OF NURSING OUTCOMES (NOC)*				
	RESULT	INDICATORS	MEASURING SCALE	TARGET SCORE	
				KEEP	INCREASE
DOMAIN: 12 COMFORT **CLASS:** 1 PHYSICAL COMFORT **CODE:** 00134 **Label (problem) (P)** Nausea **Related factors (causes) (e)** Drugs **Defining characteristics (signs and symptoms)** Nauseous sensation.	**DOMAIN:** IV HEALTH KNOWLEDGE AND BEHAVIORS **CLASS:** Q HEALTH BEHAVIOR. **CODE:1618** **EXPECTED RESULT:** CONTROL OF NAUSEA AND VOMITING	- DESCRIBES CAUSAL FACTORS - AVOIDS CAUSAL FACTORS WHEN POSSIBLE. - USES ANTIEMETIC MEDICATIONS.	1.NEVER DEMONSTRATED. 2. RARELY DEMONSTRATED. 3.SOMETIMES PROVEN. 4.FREQUENTLY DEMONSTRATED. 5.ALWAYS DEMONSTRATED.	KEEP 3 KEEP 2 KEEP 4	AUMENTA 5 AUMENTA 4 AUMENTA 4

INTERVENTIONS (NIC)	INTERVENTIONS(NIC)
MANAGEMENT OF NAUSEA 1. Assessment of nausea: duration, frequency and triggering factors. 2. Identify factors: chemotherapy medication. 3. Ensure that effective antiemetics have been administered to prevent nausea whenever possible. 4. Control environmental effects such as bad odors. 5. Encourage the patient to eat small amounts of food that are appealing to the nauseated person.	**MEDICATION MANAGEMENT.** 1. Determine which drugs are needed and administer them according to the prescribing authorization and protocol. 2. Monitor the efficacy of the medication administration modality. 3. Monitor compliance with the medication regimen.

BIBLIOGRAPHY: NANDA International 2012-2014, Moorhead, s. (2014) Nursing Outcomes Classification (NOC), Barcelona, Spain.
Elsevier., Bulechek, g. (2014) Nursing Interventions Classification (NIC), Barcelona, Spain. Elsevier.

NURSING CARE PLAN

NURSING DIAGNOSIS (NANDA)	CLASSIFICATION OF NURSING OUTCOMES (NOC)				
				TARGET SCORE	
	RESULT	INDICATORS	MEASURING SCALE	KEEP	INCREASE
DOMAIN: 11 SAFETY/PROTECTION **CLASS:** 2 PHYSICAL INJURY **CODE:** 00045 **Label (problem) (P)** Deterioration of the oral mucosa. **Related factors (causes) (e)** Side effects of chemotherapy. **Defining characteristics (signs and symptoms).** Oral ulcers and oral pain.	**DOMAIN:** FUNCTIONAL HEALTH (I) **CLASS:** SELF-CARE (D). **CODE:** 0308 **EXPECTED RESULT:** SELF-CARE: ORAL HYGIENE	- WASHES MOUTHS, THE ENCIASYLA LENGUAY MOUTHWASH.	1. SEVERELY COMPROMISED. 2. SUBSTANTIALLY COMPREMITED. 3. MODERATELY COMPROMISED. 4. SLIGHTLY COMPROMISED. 5. UNCOMMITTED.	KEEP 3	AUMENTA 4

INTERVENTIONS (NIC)	INTERVENTIONS (NIC)
RESTORATION OF ORAL HEALTH. 1. Monitor the condition of the patient's mouth, including characteristics of abnormalities. 2. Monitor changes in taste, swallowing, voice quality and comfort. 3. Obtain a physician's order to perform oral hygiene. 4. Determine the frequency needed for oral care, encouraging the patient or family to participate in scheduling or assisting with oral care as needed. 5. Instruct the patient to use a soft bristle brush or disposable mouth sponge. 6. Administer mouthwash to the patient.	**RESTORATION OF ORAL HEALTH.** 1. Apply lubricant to moisten the lips and oral mucosa. 2. Encourage patients to increase water intake. 3. Instruct the patient to avoid hot foods and liquids to prevent burns and further irritation. 4. Instruct patients on the signs and symptoms of mucositis.

BIBLIOGRAPHY: NANDA International 2012-2014, Moorhead, s. (2014) Nursing Outcomes Classification (NOC), Barcelona, Spain.
Elsevier., Bulechek, g. (2014) Nursing Interventions Classification (NIC), Barcelona, Spain. Elsevier.

NURSING CARE PLAN

NURSING DIAGNOSIS (NANDA)	CLASSIFICATION OF NURSING OUTCOMES (NOC)				
	RESULT	INDICATORS	MEASURING SCALE	TARGET SCORE KEEP	INCREASE
DOMAIN: 01 HEALTH PROMOTION. **CLASS:** 02 HEALTH MANAGEMENT. **CODE:00043** **Label (problem) (P)** Ineffective protection. **Related factors (causes) (e)** Abnormal hematologic profiles (neutropenia). **Defining characteristics (signs and symptoms)** Immune deficiency	**DOMAIN:** 02 PHYSIOLOGICAL HEALTH **CLASS:** R IMMUNE RESPONSE **CODE:** 0702 **EXPECTED RESULT:** IMMUNE STATUS	- ABSOLUTE NEUTROPHIL COUNT.	1. SEVERELY COMPROMISED. 2. SUBSTANTIALLY COMPREMITED. 3. MODERATELY COMPROMISED. 4. SLIGHTLY COMPROMISED. 5. UNCOMMITTED.	KEEP 2	AUMENTA 4

INTERVENTIONS (NIC)	INTERVENTIONS (NIC)
PROTECTION AGAINST INFECTIONS.	**PROTECTION AGAINST INFECTIONS.**
1. Observe for signs and symptoms of systemic and localized infection 2. Observe the patient's degree of vulnerability to infection. 3. Monitor the white blood cell count. Keeping in mind that if a patient is found with a neutrophil count lower than is considered severe neutropenia and isolation is required. 4. Follow the precautions for neutropenia according to the protocol of the immunohematology ward of the central military hospital, if applicable.	1. Administer an immunizing agent, if appropriate. 2. Report positive culture results to appropriate medical personnel. 3. Report suspected infections to infection control personnel. 4. Instruct the patient and family about the signs and symptoms of infection and when to report them to the nurse.
5. Limit the number of visits, if applicable. 6. Maintain asepsis standards for the patient at risk. 7. Perform isolation techniques, if necessary. 8. Record the presence of fever. 9. Teach the patient to take antibiotics as prescribed. 10. Maintain asepsis standards for the patient at risk. 11. Facilitate rest. 12. Encourage fluid intake, if appropriate. 13. Provide private room if necessary.	

BIBLIOGRAPHY: NANDA International 2012-2014, Moorhead, s. (2014) Nursing Outcomes Classification (NOC), Barcelona, Spain. Elsevier., Bulechek, g. (2014) Nursing Interventions Classification (NIC), Barcelona, Spain. Elsevier.

DIR. GRAL. EDUC. MIL. AND RECT.DE LAU.D.E.F.A. ESC. MIL. OF ENFRAS.
SEC. INV. AND DOC. MIL.

NURSING CARE PLAN					
	CLASSIFICATION OF NURSING OUTCOMES (NOC)				
	RESULT	INDICATORS	MEASURING SCALE	TARGET SCORE	
NURSING DIAGNOSIS (NANDA)				KEEP	INCREASE
DOMAIN: 01 HEALTH PROMOTION. **CLASS:** 02 HEALTH MANAGEMENT. **CODE:00043** **Label (problem) (P)** Ineffective protection. **Related factors (causes) (e)** Side effects of treatment (chemotherapy) **Defining characteristics (signs and symptoms)** Alteration of coagulation, thrombocytopenia.	**DOMAIN:** II PHYSIOLOGICAL HEALTH. **CLASS:** R IMMUNE RESPONSE **CODE:** 0409 **EXPECTED RESULT:** BLOOD COAGULATION	- PLATELET CONCENTRATION.	1. SEVERE DEVIATION FROM THE NORMAL RANGE. 2. SUBSTANTIAL DEVIATION FROM THE NORMAL RANGE. 3. MODERATE DEVIATION FROM THE NORMAL RANGE. 4. SLIGHT DEVIATION FROM THE NORMAL RANGE. 5. WITHOUT DEVIATION FROM THE NORMAL RANGE.1.	KEEP 1	AUMENTA 4
INTERVENTIONS (NIC)			**INTERVENTIONS NIC)**		

ADMINISTRATION OF BLOOD PRODUCTS.	
1. Observe or verify the patient's informed consent. 2. Verify correct patient, blood type, Rh type, unit number and expiration date and record according to hospital protocol. 3. Teach the patient the signs and symptoms of transfusion reactions (itching, dizziness, shortness of breath and chest pain). 4. Monitor the intravenous puncture site for signs of infiltration, phlebitis and local infection. 5. Monitor vital signs before, during and after transfusion.	1. Verify physician's orders 2. Obtain the patient's transfusion history. 3. Corroborate patient consent and request orders for blood product required for transfusion. 4. Verify that the blood product has been prepared, sorted and crossmatched. 5. Coordinate the return of the blood container to the laboratory after a blood reaction.
6. Observe for transfusion reactions. 7. Monitor and regulate the rate during transfusion. 8. Stop transfusion if blood reactions occur and keep veins clear with saline. 9. Refrain from administering medications or other fluids into the blood product administration routes. 10. Record the duration of the transfusion time. 11. Record the volume transfused.	

BIBLIOGRAPHY: NANDA International 2012-2014, Moorhead, s. (2014) Nursing Outcomes Classification (NOC), Barcelona, Spain. Elsevier., Bulechek, g. (2014) Nursing Interventions Classification (NIC), Barcelona, Spain. Elsevier.

DIR. GRAL. EDUC. MIL. AND RECT.DE LAU.D.E.F.A. ESC. MIL. OF ENFRAS. SEC. INV. AND DOC. MIL.

NURSING CARE PLAN					
	CLASSIFICATION OF NURSING OUTCOMES (NOC)				
				TARGET SCORE	
	RESULT	**INDICATORS**	**MEASURING SCALE**	**KEEP**	**INCREASE**
NURSING DIAGNOSIS (NANDA)					
DOMAIN: 11 SAFETY/PROTECTION **CLASS:** 2 PHYSICAL INJURY **CODE:** 00046 **Label (problem) (P)** Deterioration of skin integrity. **Related factors (causes) (e)** Radiotherapy. **Defining characteristics (signs and symptoms).** Alteration of the skin surface.	**DOMAIN:** II PHYSIOLOGICAL HEALTH. **CLASS: L** TISSUE INTEGRITY. **CODE:** 1101 **EXPECTED RESULT:** TISSUE INTEGRITY: SKIN	- INJURIES CUTANEAS	1. SERIOUS. 2. SUSTANTIAL 3. MODERATE 4. LEVE 5. NONE	KEEP 3	AUMENTA 4
INTERVENTIONS (NIC)			**INTERVENTIONS(NIC)**		

TOPICAL MEDICATION ADMINISTRATION	SKIN CARE: TOPICAL TREATMENT
1. Determine the patient's knowledge of the medication and understanding of the method of administration. 2. Determine the condition of the patient's skin in the area where the medication is applied. 3. Apply the topical drug according to this presentation. 4. Spread the medication evenly over the skin, as appropriate. 5. Teach control and self-management technique.	1. Clean with neutral or antibacterial soap. 2. Dress the patient in appropriate clothing. 3. Cover hands with gloves to check the injury.

BIBLIOGRAPHY: NANDA International 2012-2014, Moorhead, s. (2014) Nursing Outcomes Classification (NOC), Barcelona, Spain. Elsevier., Bulechek, g. (2014) Nursing Interventions Classification (NIC), Barcelona, Spain. Elsevier.

DIR. GRAL. EDUC. MIL. AND RECT.DE LAU.D.E.F.A. ESC. MIL. DE ENFRAS.SEC. INV. AND DOC. MIL.

NURSING CARE PLAN

NURSING DIAGNOSIS (NANDA)	CLASSIFICATION OF NURSING OUTCOMES (NOC)				
	RESULT	INDICATORS	MEASURING SCALE	TARGET SCORE	
				KEEP	INCREASE
DOMAIN: 4 ACTIVITY/REST **CLASS:** 1 SLEEP/REST **CODE:** 00198 **Label (problem) (P)** Sleep pattern disorder. **Related factors (causes) (e)** Lack of sleep control. **Defining characteristics (signs and symptoms)** Daytime drowsiness.	**DOMAIN: CLASS: CODE:** **EXPECTED RESULT:** DECREASED SLEEP	- HOURSFROM DREAMS FULFILLED - SLEEPS THROUGH THE NIGHT - QUALITY OF DREAM	1. SEVERELY COMPROMISED. 2. SUBSTANTIALLY COMPREMITED. 3. MODERATELY COMPROMISED. 4. SLIGHTLY COMPROMISED. 5. NO COMMITTED.	KEEP 2 KEEP 3 KEEP 3	AUMENTA 3 AUMENTA 5 AUMENTA 3

INTERVENTIONS (NIC)	INTERVENTIONSNIC)
IMPROVE SLEEP	**IMPROVE SLEEP**
1. Determine the patient's sleep/wake pattern. 2. Determine the effects of the patient's medication on sleep pattern. 3. Observe and record the number of hours of sleep of the patient. 4. Observe the psychological circumstances that alter the patient's need for rest/sleep such as fear or depression. 5. control participation in activities that cause fatigue to avoid overtiredness.	1. Encourage the patient to establish an hourly routine to avoid sleeping all the time. 2. Facilitate the maintenance of the established time routine. 3. Help the patient to limit daytime sleep by providing activities that promote wakefulness. 4. Identify the medications that the patient is taking in order to educate him/her about the effects they may cause.

BIBLIOGRAPHY: NANDA International 2012-2014, Moorhead, s. (2014) Nursing Outcomes Classification (NOC), Barcelona, Spain. Elsevier., Bulechek, g. (2014) Nursing Interventions Classification (NIC), Barcelona, Spain. Elsevier.

NURSING CARE PLAN					
	CLASSIFICATION OF NURSING OUTCOMES (NOC)				
				TARGET SCORE	
	RESULT	INDICATORS	MEASURING SCALE	KEEP	INCREASE
NURSING DIAGNOSIS (NANDA)					
DOMAIN: 5 PERCEPTION/COGNITION CLASS: 4 COGNITION **CODE:** 00161 **Label (problem) (P)** Willingness to improve their knowledge. **Defining characteristics (signs and symptoms)** Expresses interest in learning.	**DOMAIN:** V ELIGIBLE HEALTH **CLASS:** e SATISFACTION OF CARE. **CODE:** 3012. **EXPECTED RESULT:** PATIENT/USER SATISFACTION: TEACHING.	- EXPLANATION OF THE MEDICAL DIAGNOSIS. - EXPLANATION OF THE SEQUELAE EFFECTS OF THE MEDICATION.	1. NOT ENTIRELY SATISFIED. 2. SOMEWHAT SATISFIED. 3. MODERATELY SATISFIED. 4. VERY SATISFIED. 5. COMPLETELY SATISFIED.	KEEP 1 KEEP 3	AUMENTA 4 AUMENTA 5

INTERVENTIONS (NIC)	INTERVENTIONS(NIC)
FACILITATE LEARNING	**FACILITATE LEARNING**
1. Begin information only after the patient demonstrates a willingness to learn. 2. Establish realistic objective goals with the patient. 3. Identify teaching objectives clearly and in observable terms. 4. Adjust the information to the patient's level of knowledge and understanding. 5. Adjust information according to the patient's cognitive, psychomotor and/or affective abilities and disabilities. 6. Provide an environment that induces learning.	1. Establish the information in a logical sequence. 2. Relate the information to the patient's personal wants/needs. 3. Provide information that is appropriate to the patient's values and beliefs. 4. Use familiar language. 5. Provide information in a stimulating way. 6. Allow adequate time to master the content. 7. Repeat important information. 8. Correct misinterpretations of information, if applicable.

BIBLIOGRAPHY: NANDA International 2012-2014, Moorhead, s. (2014) Nursing Outcomes Classification (NOC), Barcelona, Spain. Elsevier., Bulechek, g. (2014) Nursing Interventions Classification (NIC), Barcelona, Spain. Elsevier.

NURSING CARE PLAN					
NURSING DIAGNOSIS (NANDA)	*CLASSIFICATION OF NURSING OUTCOMES (NOC)*				
	RESULT	INDICATORS	MEASURING SCALE	TARGET SCORE	
				KEEP	INCREASE
DOMAIN: 8 SEXUALITY **CLASS:** 2 SEXUAL FUNCTION. **CODE:** 00065 **Label (problem) (P)** Ineffective sexual pattern. **Related factors (causes) (e)** Poor knowledge of disease-related responses and medical treatment. **Defining characteristics (signs and symptoms)** Expresses changes in sexual behaviors.	**DOMAIN:** IV KNOWLEDGE OF SEXUAL BEHAVIOR **CLASS:**S HEALTH KNOWLEDGE. **CODE:** 1815 **EXPECTED RESULT:** KNOWLEDGE: SEXUAL FUNCTIONING.	CHANGES IN KNOWLEDGE AB OUT THE SEXUALITY. KNOWLEDGE OF THE REPRODUCTION.	1. NO KNOWLEDGE. 2. KNOWLEDGE IS SCARCE. 3. MODERATE KNOWLEDGE. 4. KNOWLEDGE. 5. EXTENSIVE KNOWLEDGE.	KEEP 1 KEEP 1	AUMENTA 4 AUMENTA 4
INTERVENTIONS (NIC)			**INTERVENTIONSNIC)**		

SEXUAL COUNSELING

1. Establish a therapeutic relationship based on trust and respect.
2. Provide privacy and ensure confidentiality.
3. Explain to the patient at the beginning of the relationship that sexuality is an important part of life and that illness and medications often disrupt sexual functioning.
4. Encourage the patient to verbalize fears and ask questions about sexual functioning.
5. Collect the patient's sexual history paying attention to the terms used by the patient to describe sexual function.

SEXUAL COUNSELING

1. Discuss the effects of health and illness on sexuality.
2. Comment on the effect of the medication.
3. Helping the patient to express grief and anger about alterations in functioning.
4. Use humor and encourage the patient to use humor to relieve anxiety and embarrassment, with gentleness and respect for the patient's beliefs and culture.
5. Refer the patient to sex therapy, when appropriate.

BIBLIOGRAPHY: NANDA International 2012-2014, Moorhead, s. (2014) Nursing Outcomes Classification (NOC), Barcelona, Spain. Elsevier., Bulechek, g. (2014) Nursing Interventions Classification (NIC), Barcelona, Spain. Elsevier.

DIR. GRAL. EDUC. MIL. EDUC
RECTOR OF THE U.D.E.F.A.

. MIL. OF ENFRAS.
SEC. INV. AND DOC. MIL.

NURSING CARE PLAN					
	CLASSIFICATION OF NURSING OUTCOMES (NOC)				
	RESULT	INDICATORS	MEASURING SCALE	TARGET SCORE	
				KEEP	INCREASE
NURSING DIAGNOSIS (NANDA)					
DOMAIN: 12 COMFORT. **CLASS:** 1 COMFORT. **CODE:** 00214. **Label (problem) (P)** Discomfort. **Related factors (causes) (e)** Disease-related symptoms and side effects of treatment. **Defining characteristics (signs and symptoms).** Expresses lack of calmness in the situation, sighs, fear and anxiety.	**DOMAIN:** V PERCEIVED HEALTH. **CLASS:** V SYMPTOMATOLOGY. **CODE:** 2103. **EXPECTED RESULT:** SEVERITY OF SYMPTOMS	- DISCOMFORT ASSOCIATED WITH THE SYMPTOM.	1. SERIOUS. 2. SUBSTANTIAL. 3. MODERATE. 4. MILD. 5. NONE.	KEEP 2	AUMENTA 4
INTERVENTIONS (NIC)			**INTERVENTIONSNIC)**		
INCREASE SUPPORT SYSTEMS. 1. Estimate the psychological response to the situation and the availability of the support system. 2. Determine the suitability of existing social networks. 3. Determine the degree of family and financial support, as well as other resources. 4. Provide services with an appreciative and supportive attitude. 5. Involve the family in the care and planning.			**DECREASE IN ANXIETY.** 1. Clearly establish expectations for patient behavior. 2. Explain all procedures, including possible sensations to be experienced during the procedure. 3. Provide objective information regarding diagnosis, treatment and prognosis. 4. Listen carefully. 5. Help the patient identify situations that precipitate anxiety. 6. Support with adequate defense mechanisms.		

BIBLIOGRAPHY: NANDA International 2012-2014, Moorhead, s. (2014) Nursing Outcomes Classification (NOC), Barcelona, Spain. Elsevier., Bulechek, g. (2014) Nursing Interventions Classification (NIC), Barcelona, Spain. Elsevier.

DIR. GRAL. EDUC. MIL. AND RECT.DE LAU.D.E.F.A.

NURSING CARE PLAN

NURSING DIAGNOSIS (NANDA)	CLASSIFICATION OF NURSING OUTCOMES (NOC)				
	RESULT	INDICATORS	MEASURING SCALE	TARGET SCORE	
				KEEP	INCREASE
DOMAIN: 11 SECURITY/PROTECTION **CLASS:** 02 PHYSICAL INJURY. **CODE:00206** **Label (problem) (P)** Risk of bleeding. **Related factors (causes) (e)** Side effects of chemotherapy and thrombocytopenia.	**DOMAIN:** IV HEALTH KNOWLEDGE AND BEHAVIOR. **CLASS:** T RISK CONTROL AND SAFETY. **CODE:** 1902. **EXPECTED RESULT:** RISK CONTROL	- RECOGNIZES RISK FACTORS. - AVOID EXPOSURE TO HEALTH THREATS.	1.NEVER DEMONSTRATED. 2.RARELY DEMONSTRATED. 3.SOMETIMES PROVEN. 4.FREQUENTLY DEMONSTRATED. 5.ALWAYS DEMONSTRATED.	KEEP 2 KEEP 2	AUMENTA 4 AUMENTA 4

INTERVENTIONS (NIC)	INTERVENTIONSNIC)
CHEMOTHERAPY MANAGEMENT 1. Provide information to the patient and family about how antineoplastic drugs work, side effects of chemotherapy and bone marrow function. 2. Inform the patient and family to immediately report fever, nosebleeds, excessive bruising and dark colored stools.	**BLEEDING PREVENTION** 1. Monitor the patient closely for bleeding. 2. Protect the patient from traumas that may cause bleeding: arrange the furniture in such a way that he/she will not trip and bruise himself/herself with it, eliminate the accumulation of objects on the floor. Avoid wearing very tight clothing or any buttons that may injure the skin. Do not lift heavy objects.
3. Control of laboratory tests to know the values of platelets that the patient has.	3. Use soft toothbrushes in oral hygiene, ambulation with footwear, use electric razor instead of razor blade.

BIBLIOGRAPHY: NANDA International 2012-2014, Moorhead, s. (2014) Nursing Outcomes Classification (NOC), Barcelona, Spain. Elsevier., Bulechek, g. (2014) Nursing Interventions Classification (NIC), Barcelona, Spain. Elsevier.

j. Description of the evaluation instrument.

Plans are elaborated by nursing diagnoses and evaluated with the Likert scale to assess whether or not the results shown with respect to the improvement of the needs of the patient with non-Hodgkin's lymphoma were favorable or not. The interventions suitable for the achievement of objectives are selected from a codified list taking Henderson as a reference, selecting those activities in which the patient can also participate.

The Likert scale is graduated from 1 to 5; if the indicator does not change, it remains at 0, i.e. it neither increases nor decreases. The indicators generate a corresponding change variable, each indicator being evaluated as follows:

+   2 = worsens 2 points at discharge with respect to admission.

+   1 = worsens 1 point at discharge with respect to admission.

   0 = does not vary.

+   1=   improvement of 1   point with respect to income.

+   2=   improvement of 2 points with respect   to income .

+   3=   improvement of 3 points with respect   to income .

+   4=   improvement of 4 points with respect   to income .

The benefit or worsening for each of the altered nursing diagnoses, from the moment of application and that assigned at the end of the application, are evaluated by adding or subtracting the respective scales, constituting the indicators of improvement or worsening as previously described.

The indicator analyzed in the nursing care plans (PLACE) is the improvement/improvement observed by the difference in the value of the scale evaluated at admission and at the end of the application of the Nursing Care Process. The evaluation of nursing diagnoses is as follows:

Chapter 3

III. RESULTS

Taking into account the objective of the process, which is to evaluate the improvement of the side effects of chemotherapy after the application of a Nursing Care Process to a patient with non-Hodgkin's lymphoma, the following analysis of results is carried out.

From Monday, February 15 to February 26, 2016, for a total of 10 working days, the Nursing Care Process was applied to a male patient who met the inclusion criteria, age 20 years, active military, musician, diagnosed in January 2015 with non-Hodgkin's lymphoma, originally from Oaxaca, single marital status with no offspring, currently undergoing chemotherapy and radiotherapy treatment, according to the assessment instrument of the theorist Virginia Henderson the following most affected needs are observed "nutrition, safety, skin protection, communication, rest and sleep, and learning".

1. The patient's nutrition is detected as the first need, for which two labels are diagnosed: "Nutritional imbalance and, Nausea"; to obtain a result it is achieved to set a goal with the patient to increase the income of the foods that are given to him suggesting expressing which foods are not to his liking to the dietitian, performing the convenient interventions to reduce nausea, and the change of the first indicator from substantial to mild and the second indicator changing from moderate to mild is obtained, which shows an improvement with respect to the admission and the tenth day of the application.

2. Regarding the need for hygiene and skin protection, the following are diagnosed: "Impairment of the oral mucosa and Impairment of skin integrity", with the perseverance of the interventions described in the place it is possible to change the indicators of the first diagnosis from moderately

compromised to slightly compromised and of the second diagnosis from moderately to mild respectively , demonstrating an improvement.

3. The altered need for safety is observed with regard to the diagnoses related to ineffective protection, the indicator *"absolute neutrophil count"* remains substantially compromised and the indicator *"platelet concentration"* in a severe deviation to the normal range, so emphasis is placed on nursing interventions and activities to reduce the degree of affection, presenting an improvement of slightly compromised for the first indicator and a slight deviation to the normal range of the second indicator, which shows the improvement of the need.

4. Analyzing Virginia Henderson's fifth need "rest and sleep", the label "sleep disorder" is detected, showing an improvement in the change of indicator one from substantially compromised to moderately compromised with an improvement, indicator two from moderately to not compromised and indicator three with respect to sleep quality does not vary, remaining at moderately compromised.

5. The diagnosis that represents the fourteenth need that demands to study, discover or satisfy the curiosity that leads to a normal development of health is: *Willingness to improve their knowledge manifested by expressed interest in learning,* successfully increasing the indicators from *not at all satisfied* to *very satisfied*; and, *from somewhat satisfied* to *very satisfied*, with respect to income. It is worth mentioning that the patient was given two informative leaflets about his disease and the recommendations regarding the side effects of chemotherapy, thus achieving the patient's satisfaction and interest in obtaining more information using the Internet, electronic devices and social networks with the aim of improving his general health conditions. (APPENDIX D)

6. The confirmation of obtaining improvement with respect to the need for communication with the diagnosis: "Ineffective sexual pattern", was a difficult challenge since it was expected to be able to transmit the appropriate information in a simple and satisfactory manner, managing to obtain the patient's trust, an improvement is obtained with respect to the admission, changing the indicator from no knowledge to substantial knowledge.

7. The last diagnosis was aimed at improving the discomfort related to the disease and side effects of the treatment, interventions were sought to contribute to the success in improving the indicator, which changed from substantial to mild, obtaining improvement with respect to income.

Given the above findings, it is demonstrated that nursing interventions produce a favorable evolution towards the improvement of the patient's needs according to the Virginia Henderson model, which were altered on admission. Considering the above information, the significant improvement in the objectives (NOC) of the PLACES can be observed, adding up to a positive result.

Chapter 4

IV. DISCUSSION

Although Marriner establishes that nursing care started from the existence of a stage called domestic, in which she mentions that women were in charge of home care without any scientific basis, with the sole purpose of maintaining life, it was not until the middle of the 19th century that Nightengale gave them a scientific character.

From that time to the present, different theoretical models have emerged that have conceptualized the different ways of organizing care, for which this Nursing Care Process uses the assessment of Virginia Henderson covering her metaparadigm care, environment and person and that according to Alligood this theorist exhorts the nursing functions in which we must not only assess the needs but also the conditions and the pathological states that alter it, for which I fully agree.

Every discipline needs a standardized language that clearly defines a conceptual framework of the needs we wish to address in the patient, so Bulechek in the Nursing Intervention Classification (NIC) book outlines the importance of nursing interventions: complete, research-based, based on existing practice, reflects current clinical practice and research, simple structure, clear language and clinical meaning, stable structure and process of continuous improvement, subject to field testing, accessible and are related to other classifications such as NANDA and NOC, in my opinion, allows to have a conceptual basis and a specific epistemology that allows the study and transmission of knowledge in the nursing area.

Said by Moran, the process is the application of the scientific resolution of nursing care problems following a certain method. To complement the previous concept, we will mention that the process implies a series of knowledge on the use of the NANDA, NIC, NOC taxonomies and that the planning of nursing care is an essential instrument to structure evidence-based nursing.

CONCLUSION

Subsequent to the data analysis, it can be concluded that the patient expresses his satisfaction with the nursing interventions provided and for participating in this research project, he expresses that the process provided him with a relationship of trust with the subscriber, he feels more comfortable, included, informed, anticipated and with the ability to follow up on his illness.

With respect to the observed altered needs of the patient, a notorious change is achieved since the basis of the nursing care process was strictly selected with the objective of improving the side effects of chemotherapy in the patient.

The main difficulty of the nursing staff observed is the lack of familiarity with the nursing care process due to the absence of the application in the Central Military Hospital where the application was carried out. What is noteworthy to mention is that the nursing staff has clear and precise information on the situation of the patient, his family or relatives, which supports the reliability and good communication that exists between health professionals and patients.

RECOMMENDATIONS

Based on the National Health System and based on the analysis of this process, the following recommendations can be suggested.

1. To encourage the future application of the Nursing Care Process at the Central Military Hospital as written evidence of the nursing profession.
2. To take the present Nursing Care Process as a basis for creating evidence-based and standardized Nursing Care Plans that allow nursing care to the patient with non-Hodgkin's Lymphoma in the Immunohematology ward and thus contribute to the patient's well-being.
3. Include the use of NANDA, NIC, NOC taxonomies in the daily practice of nursing staff for familiarization.
4. To perform continuous studies to patients to whom a Nursing Care Process is applied in order to evaluate the improvement of the patient and the benefit achieved.
5. Promote a common language between nurses who know the Nursing Care Process and those who do not, in order to share knowledge and experience.

BIBLIOGRAPHY

1. Alfaro (2010). *Application of the Nursing Process.* Spain: Linpiccot.

2. Alligood, M. R. (2007). *Models and Theories in Nursing.* Madrid, Spain: Elsevier.

3. Arguelles, G. J. (2009). *Fundamentals of Hematology.* United States: Panamericana.

4. Avila, G. (2001). *Frequent medical disorders in oncology.* Mexico: Graw Hill Interamericana.

5. Cavanagh, S. J. (2006). *Models of Nursing.* Pennsylvania: Scientific and Technological Editions.

6. Dermot (2010). *Cancer.* Madrid: Wolters Kluwer.

7. Fernandez, A. A. (2005). *Terapia de oncohematologia.* Madrid: Elsevier.

8. Fry (2010). *Ethics in Nursing Practice .* Madrid, Spain: Manual Moderno.

9. Hillman, a. r. (2006). *Hematology in clinical practice.* Mexico, D.F.: Mc Graw-Hill.

10. Lanuza; et, al. (2008). *Aplicacion de Modelos a la Enfemería.* Bogota, Colombia: Elsevier.

11. Marriner, r. (2004). *el proceso de atencion de enfermeria.* mexico, d.f.: el manual moderno.

12. Moran (2010). *Nursing Process.* Mexico City: Trillas.

13. NOM-022-SSA3-2012. *(2012). For the administration of infusion therapy.*

14. NOM-045-SSA2-2005 *(2005). For epidemiological surveillance, prevention or control of nosocomial infections.*

15. Reyes, E. (2015). *Fundamentos de Enfermería.* México, D.F.: Manual Moderno.

16. Terry, C. L., & Wuaver, A. (2012). *Nursing: Cancer care.* Spain: Manual Moderno.

17. Secretary of Health, (2009). *Guía de Practica Clínica, Linfomas No Hodgkin en el Adulto,* Centro Nacional de Excelencia Tecnológica en Salud.

ANNEXES

ANNEX A

VIRGINIA HENDERSON'S "BASIC NEEDS" MODEL CLINICAL NURSING ASSESSMENT

GENERAL DATA

DATE:	TIME:	FR:
NAME:		FC:
SEX:	AGE:	TA:
ADDRESS:		TEMP:
DIAGNOSIS:		WEIGHT: / SIZE:
REASON FOR ADMISSION:		OCCUPATION:
		ESTADOCIVIL:

1. BASIC NEED FOR OXYGENATION

RESPIRATORY RATE:	CHARACTERISTICS OF LUNG SOUNDS	NORMAL	ALTERATIONS	TOS	YES
		SIBILANTS	ASSOCIATED PAIN BREATHING		
		ESTERNOTES	NASAL ALETEUS		NO
		PROLONGED	INTERCOSTAL PULL		

TOS SINO	COUGH TYPE: N/A	DYSNEA	DOES NOT PRESENT
	PAROXISTICS		OCCASIONALLY
	WITH SPUTO		HABITUAL
	HEMOPTISIS		EACH PHYSICAL ACTIVITY
	SECA		WHEN SLEEPING

CYANOSIS		CHARACTERISTICS OF RESPIRATION:		THORACIC DEFORMITIES	
	DOES NOT PRESENT		RITMICA		DOES NOT PRESENT
	CENTRAL		BRADIPNEA		PIGEON THORAX
	PERIPHERAL		TAQUIPNEA		FUNNEL THORAX
	ENTEROGENEA		OTHER		OTHERS:

SMOKING: SINO	CIGARETTES PER DAY:		AGE AT WHICH HE STARTED SMOKING:	

HISTORY OF CARDIORESPIRATORY DISEASES: ASTHMA   TACHYCARDIAPRECORDIAL PAIN

2. BASIC NUTRITIONAL AND HYDRATION NEEDS

No. OF MEALS PER DIA:	FOOD ALLERGIES:		APPETITE IN THE HOSPITAL	NORMAL	DIET TYPE:	
				INCREASED	AMOUNT OF LIQUIDS INGESTED:	
				DECREASED		

DIFFICULTY IN SWALLOWING:	NONE	NASOGASTRIC TUBE	CONTRAINDICATED FOODS:	
	TO SWALLOW SOLIDS	DOES NOT TOLERATE DIET		
	TO SWALLOW LIQUIDS	REFLUX		
	NAUSEA	OTHER	SUPPLEMENTS:	

SIGNS OF MALNUTRITION	NONE	HAIR LOSS	COMPLETE DENTURE	YES	ALCOHOL CONSUMPTION	YES
	PALE	DRY HAIR		NO		NO
	DRY AND SCALY SKIN	MUSCULAR HYPOTONIA	CARIES	ULCERAS ORALS	FREQUENCY: N/A	
	MUSCLE SPASMS	EDEMA	GUM INFLAMMATION		PAIN	PIROSIS
			DIGESTIVE DISORDERS:		ACIDITY	EMESIS
					FLATULENCIES	OTHER

WEIGHT LOSS:					
	YES	NO	BMI:	WEIGHT:	SIZE:
PREFERENCES OR DISLIKES:					
REMARKS:					

3. BASIC NEED FOR DISPOSAL

NUMBER OF EVACUATIONS:	CHARACTERISTICS				NONE	AID:
	YELLOW:	DIARRHEA	STRENGTH	ALTERATIONS:	STRENGTH	ENEMAS
	GREEN:	PASTOSA	HEMORROIDS		HEMORROIDS	FOOD
	COFFEE:	LIQUID	INCONTINENCE		INCONTINENCE	MEDICATIONS
	BLACK:	SEMILIQUID	OTHERS:		OTHERS:	LIQUIDS
REMARKS:						

URINARIA

URINATION PER DAY:	CHARACTERISTICS			NONE	HEMATURIA	ENEURESIS
	CLARA	NO ODOR		TENESMO	ANURIA	
	YELLOW	WITH THE SMELL OF MEDICINE	ALTERATIONS	DISURIA	ESCOZOR	OTHERS:
	PARDA					
	CONCENTRATED	OTHER		NICTURIA	POLYACHIURIA	

AXIAL DIMENSIONS	INTERMITTENT PROBING	COVER	NONE
	PERMANENT PROBING	OTHER	

GENITALS			REMARKS:	
ALTERATIONS:		TYPE OF ALTERATION:		
YES	NO	ERUPTIONS	SECRETIONS	IRRITATION

4. MOVE AND MAINTAIN GOOD POSTURE

MOVEMENTS	AUTONOMOUS		LIMITATIONS IN AMBULATION.	CANE	ALTERATIONS	
	ASSISTED WALKING OR SITTING			FINE	FATIGUE	DECUBITUS ULCERS:
	RELATIVE IN BED			WALKER	WEAKNESS	
				WHEELCHAIR	JOINT STIFFNESS:	PARESTHESIA
	ABSOLUTE REST			NONE		PAIN
POSITION	DC. DORSAL	DC. VENTRAL	DC. RIGHT SIDE.	DC. LEFT SIDE	SEMIFOWLER	FOWLER
HYGIENIC MEASURES WHEN MOVING		YES	NO	KEEP		SINO
PHYSICAL EXERCISE		YES	NO	TYPE OF FISCAL YEAR:		ASSETSLIABILITIES

5. BASIC NEED FOR REST AND SLEEP

HOURS OF DREAM A DAY:	ALTERATIONS			USE OF VOLTAGE REDUCERS:	PHARMACOTICS
14 HOURS				SINO	
	INSOMNIA	HYPERSOMNIA	NIGHTMARES		HERBOLARIA

	SOMNOLENCE	NIGHT SWEAT	ANXIETY		MASSAGE
	FEAR	DIFFICULTY IN BREATHE	PAIN		MUSIC
REMARKS:					READING

6. BASIC NEED TO WEAR APPROPRIATE CLOTHING					
ACCEPTS HOSPITAL LINEN	YES	NO	**WEAR SPECIAL CLOTHING**	YES	NO
DIFFICULTY DRESSING	YES	NO	**ALIÑO**	ADEQUATE	INADEQUATE
FINANCIAL RESOURCES TO WEAR CLEAN CLOTHES:				YES	NO

7'. BASIC NEED FOR THERMOREGULATION					
SITE OF TOMA:	AXILAR	VAGINAL	**ALTERATIONS:**	**PROTECTION AGAINST TEMPERATURE CHANGES**	
	RECTAL	INGUINAL	HYPERTHERMIA COLD SKIN	YES	NO
	BUCAL	OTHER	HYPOTHERMIA SCALOSPHROSPHROS		
			NIGHT SWEATS		
REMARKS:					

8. BASIC NEED FOR SKIN HYGIENE AND PROTECTION					
BATH		YES	SELF-EMPLOYED		HEMATOMAS
AUTONOMOUS	**HAIR WASHING**	NO	ASSISTED		CICATRIES
ASSISTED	**ORAL HYGIENE**	YES	SELF-EMPLOYED	**SKIN ALTERATIONS:**	SKIN DEHYDRATION
OF SPONGE		NO	ASSISTED		
HAND WASHING		YES	NO		DESCAMATION
ALTERATIONS OF THE ORAL MUCOSA:		MUCOSITIS	STOMATITIS	GINGIVORRAGIA	ODONTALGIA	GINGIVITIS
REMARKS:					

9. NEED FOR SAFETY AND SECURITY					
STATE OF ALERTNESS:	ALERT		**INSULATION:**	YES	**TYPE OF INSULATION:**
	ORIENTED			NO	
	CONSIENTE	**DRUG ALLERGY:**	**RISK OF FALLING:**	YES	**SECURITY MEASURES:**	MEDICATION
	SLEEP			NO		BARANDALES
	STUPOR		**SURVEILLANCE**	YES		FASTENERS
	COMA			NO		OTHERS:

HABITS THAT AFFECT PERSONAL SAFETY:	CHARACTERISTICS THAT CONSTITUTE A HAZARD IN YOUR HOME:		HEALTH RISKS:	

10. BASIC NEED FOR COMMUNICATION AND SEXUALITY					

LANGUAGE: DIALECT:	ALTERATIONS				ADDITMENTS	APPARATUS AUDITORY:
	AFASIA	SIGN COMMUNICATION		MENTAL ILLNESS		
	DISERTRY	MUDEZ	MUTISM			
	DEAFNESS	TARTAMUDEZ	NONE	INSULATION		LENSES:

DOES IT COUNT AS WORK TO EXPRESS YOUR FEELINGS ABOUT YOUR CONDITION? WHY?		DO YOU ASK FOR HELP WHEN YOU NEED IT?	
THE RELATIONSHIP IS YOUR FAMILY IS:	GOOD	MALA	REGULAR
INITIATION OF SEXUAL RELATIONS:	USES A CONTRACEPTIVE METHOD:		
YOUR CURRENT SEXUAL ACTIVITY HAS:	INCREASED	NORMAL	DECREASED
FEELINGS OR SITUATIONS THAT AFFECT THEIR SEXUALITY:			

11. BASIC NEED FOR BELIEFS AND VALUES				
RELIGION		IS YOUR RELIGION IMPORTANT TO YOU?		DO YOU HAVE CONFLICTS BETWEEN YOUR BELIEFS AND HEALTH ISSUES?
CATHOLIC	CHRISTIAN			
JEHOVAH'S WITNESS	MORMONS	YES	NO	
OTHER:		SPECIAL (RELIGIOUS) REQUESTS:		

12. BASIC NEED FOR WORK AND SELF-FULFILLMENT	
PREVIOUS EMPLOYMENT:	ANXIETY ABOUT EMPLOYMENT DUE TO ILLNESS?
CURRENT EMPLOYMENT:	ECONOMIC DISTRESS?
ACTIVITIES YOU WOULD LIKE TO DO:	

13. BASIC NEED FOR SELF-FULFILLMENT.					
ACTIVITIES YOU WOULD LIKE TO DO:	FAVORITE ACTIVITIES			FACTORS THAT MAKE IT DIFFICULT FOR THEM TO BE DISTRACTED WHILE HOSPITALIZED:	PAIN
	READ	SPORTS	PLATICAR		WEAKNESS
	LISTEN TO MUSIC	WALK	SURFING THE INTERNET		ANGUSTIA

<table>
<tr><td rowspan="2">REMARKS:</td><td></td><td>PLAY CARDS</td><td>TRAVEL</td><td rowspan="2"></td><td>DEPRESSION</td></tr>
<tr><td>CHESS</td><td>SLEEP</td><td>DANCE</td><td>SOLEDAD</td></tr>
</table>

	14. BASIC LEARNING NEEDS.			

ACADEMIC LEVEL		ARE YOU INTERESTED IN LEARNING ABOUT YOUR DISEASE?			
ANALPHABET	PREPARATORY	YES		NO	
PRIMARY	UNIVERSITY	HOW WOULD YOU RATE YOUR NURSING KNOWLEDGE?			
SECONDARY	MAESTRIA	NULO	POCO	REGULAR	SUFFICIENT
REMARKS:					

SECRETARIAT OF NATIONAL DEFENSE

DIR. GRAL. EDUC. MIL. EDUC
RECT. OF THE U.D.E.E.F.A.F.A.
DOC. MIL.

. MIL. OF ENFRAS.
SEC. INV. AND

Need	Objective data	Subjective data
Oxygenation.		
Nutrition and Hydration.		
Elimination.		
Moving and maintaining good posture.		
Rest and Sleep.		
Use of Appropriate Clothing.		
Thermoregulation.		
Skin Hygiene and Protection.		
Avoid Dangers.		
Communication and Sexuality.		
Living according to Values and Beliefs.		
T rabajar y Realizarse.		
Participate in recreational activities.		
Learning.		

ANNEX C
REQUIREMENTS PRIORITIZATION

Need	Objective data	Subjective data
Oxygenation.		
Nutrition and Hydration.		
Elimination.		
Moving and maintaining good posture.		
Rest and Sleep.		
Use of Appropriate Clothing.		
Thermoregulation.		
Skin Hygiene and Protection.		
Avoid Dangers.		
Communication and Sexuality.		
Living according to Values and Beliefs.		
Work and fulfillment.		
Participate in recreational activities.		
Learning.		

ANNEX D

SECRETARIAT OF NATIONAL DEFENSE

DIR. GRAL. EDUC. MIL. AND RECTOR.OF LAU.D.E.F.A.

NURSING CARE PLAN					
NURSING DIAGNOSIS (NANDA)	*CLASSIFICATION OF NURSING OUTCOMES (NOC)*			TARGET SCORE	
	RESULT	INDICATORS	MEASURING SCALE	KEEP	INCREASE
DOMAIN: CLASS: CODE: Label (problem) (P) Related factors (causes) (e) Defining characteristics (signs and symptoms).	DOMAIN: CLASS: CODE: EXPECTED RESULT:				
INTERVENTIONS (NIC)	INTERVENTIONS NIC)				
BIBLIOGRAPHY:					

¿QUE ES LA QUIMIOTERAPIA?

Es un tratamiento que utiliza una gran variedad de fármacos que tienen la finalidad de atacar a las células malignas pero también afectan algunas células sanas lo que causa en usted algunos síntomas de malestar.

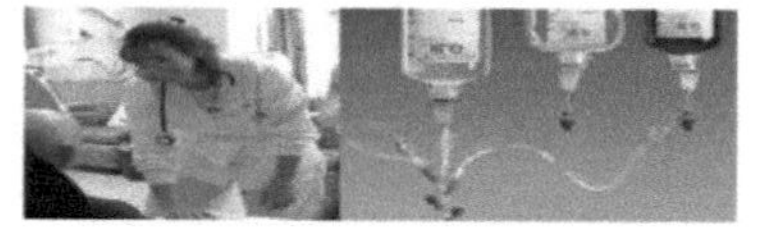

ALGUNOS EFECTOS DE LA QUIMIOTERAPIA

- Acumulación de líquido o linfedema.
- Afecciones cutáneas, deshidratación, edema o retención de líquidos.
- Anemia.
- Caída del cabello o alopecia.
- Cambios en el gusto.
- Confusión mental o delirio.
- Diarrea.
- Dificultad para respirar o disnea.
- Dolores de cabeza.
- Efectos secundarios sobre el sistema nervioso.
- Estreñimiento, fatiga e infección.
- Pérdida de peso, pérdida de apetito, náuseas y vomito.
- Problemas de coagulación.
- Problemas del sueño: hipersomnia, somnolencia o insomnio.

ANEXO E
RECOMENDACIONES PARA MANEJAR LOS EVENTOS ADVERSOS DE LA QUIMITERAPIA

CANSANCIO Y FATIGA

Es probable que se sienta cansado por lo que es recomendable utilice su energía para actividades importantes, practique ejercicios como yoga, tai-chi y estiramiento esto le ayudara a relajarse ya disminuir su estrés. El ejercicio solo con indicación médica.

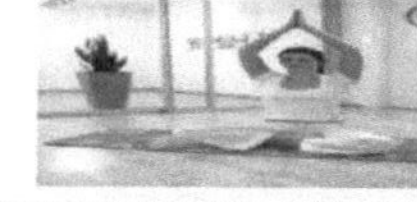

ALTERACIONES EN EL SENTIDO DEL GUSTO.

Procure comer alimentos con poco condimento, olores y aspectos agradables. Sustituya sus cubiertos habituales por unos de plástico.

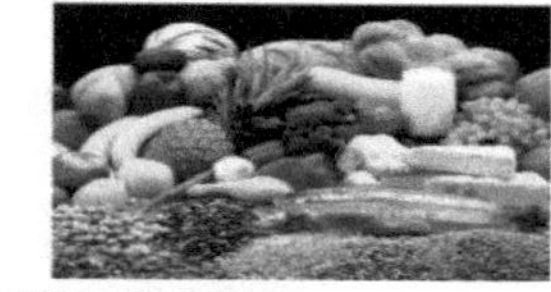

NAUSEAS Y VOMITO

Bebe muchos líquidos para evitar la deshidratación por el vómito. Coma 3-4 horas antes de la quimioterapia y evite comidas pesadas y con mucha grasa. Trate de salir a tomar aire fresco

PERDIDA DE PESO.

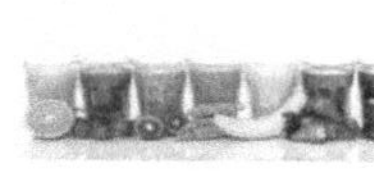

Es normal que baje de peso por la quimioterapia por lo cual debe tratar de comer bien se recomienda caminar media hora antes de cada comida para aumentar su apetito, comer acompañado, escuchando música o viendo la televisión. Las frutas y verduras que ingiera deberán estar desinfectadas y hervidas para evitar riesgos de infecciones.

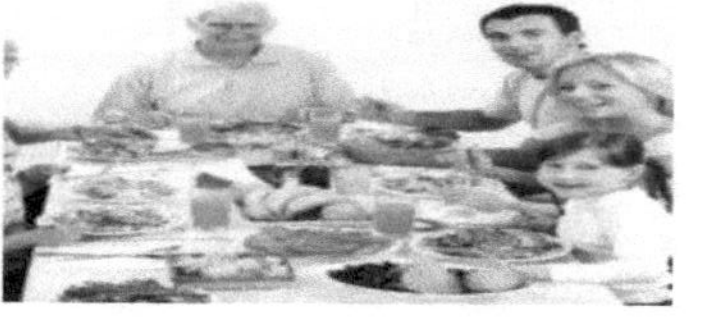

DIARREA.

Pasadas dos o tres horas del inicio de la diarrea beba pequeños sorbos de agua cada 10 minutos a lo largo del día. Evite tomar lácteos y elimine irritantes como el café y alcohol.

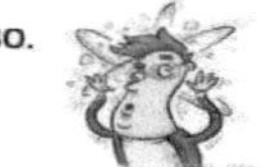

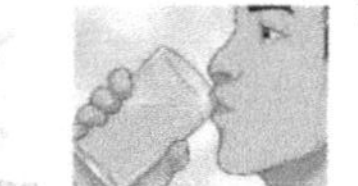

ESTREÑIMIENTO.

Coma alimentos con fibra y abundante agua. No se quede con las ganas de ir al baño.

DIFICULTAD RESPIRATORIA

Practique ejercicios de respiración abdominal y posturas en las que sienta que respira mejor.

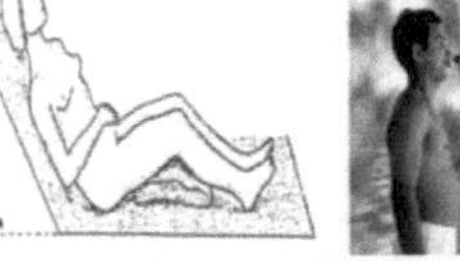

RIESGO DE INFECCIONES.

Lave sus manos antes de comer y de preparar sus alimentos. Evite contacto con mascotas. Evite alimentos crudos y prefiera la fruta pelada. Utilice cubrebocas al salir a la calle, no saludе besos a las personas y evite ir a lugares concurridos y a personas con gripe o tos.

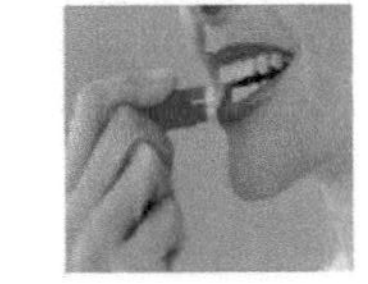

IRRITACION EN LAPIEL.

Lave su piel con agua y jabón suave. Seque su piel con pequeños toques. Utilice ropa poco ajuntada y de fibras suaves. Evite tomar el sol sin tratamiento contra los rayos UV.

PERDIDA DE CABELLO

Es inevitable la pérdida de cabello por lo que es recomendable el uso de sombreros, gorros

o pañueletas o pelucas de su preferencia. Puede utilizar el shampo y acondicionador que prefiera.

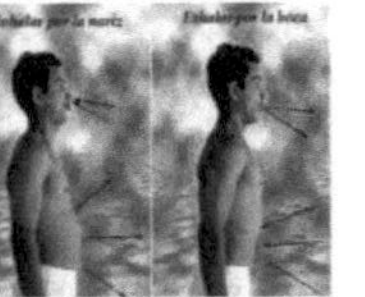

ULCERAS EN LA BOCA (AFTAS)

Enjuague su boca y lubrique sus labios antes de comer. Tome líquidos durante todo el día. Evite alimentos muy fríos, calientes o duros. Enjuague con bicarbonato la boca para aliviar el dolor.

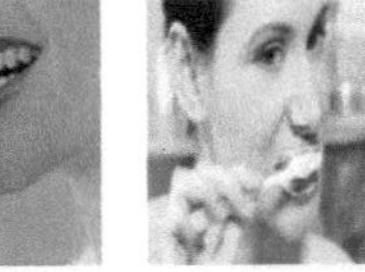

En caso de fiebre, hemorragia o dolor no se automedique acuda de inmediato al doctor.

SALA DE INMUHEMATOLOGIA.
Realizo: Cdte. 4° Año América Hernández Robles.

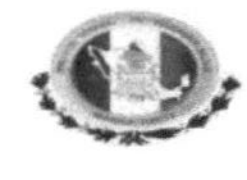
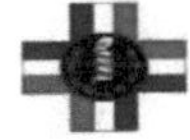
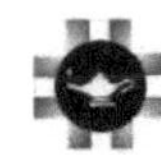

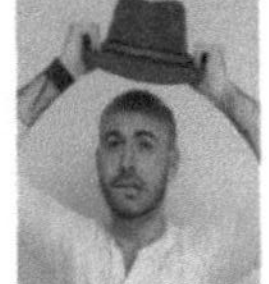

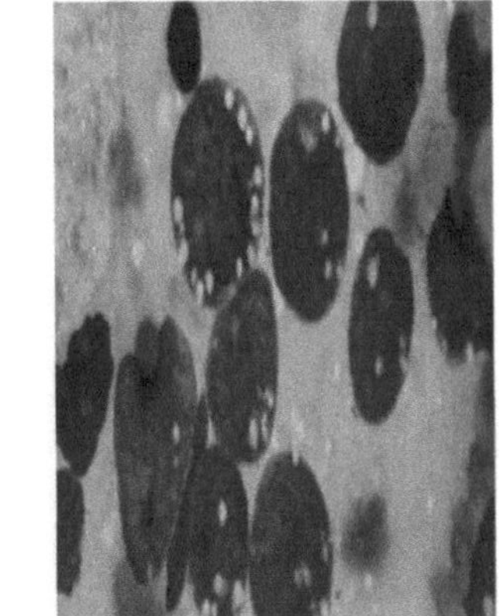

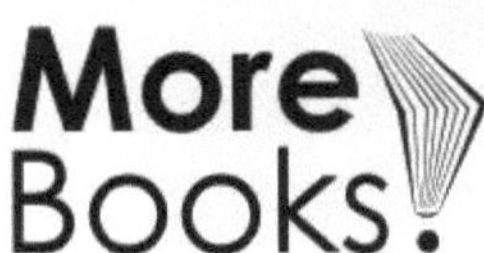

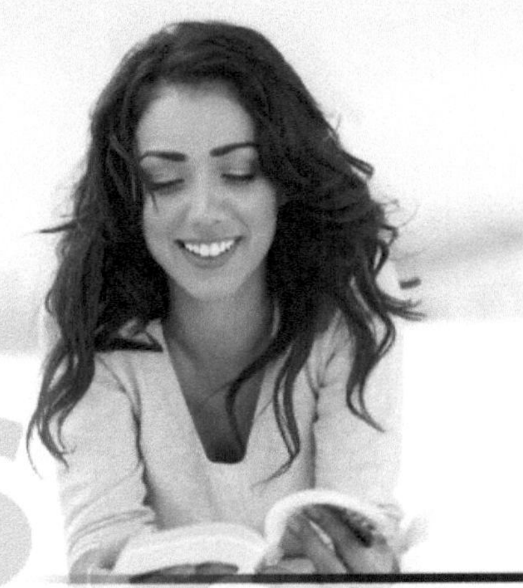

yes
I want morebooks!

Buy your books fast and straightforward online - at one of world's fastest growing online book stores! Environmentally sound due to Print-on-Demand technologies.

Buy your books online at
www.morebooks.shop

Kaufen Sie Ihre Bücher schnell und unkompliziert online – auf einer der am schnellsten wachsenden Buchhandelsplattformen weltweit! Dank Print-On-Demand umwelt- und ressourcenschonend produzi ert.

Bücher schneller online kaufen
www.morebooks.shop

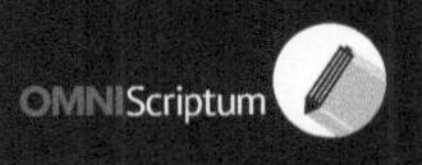

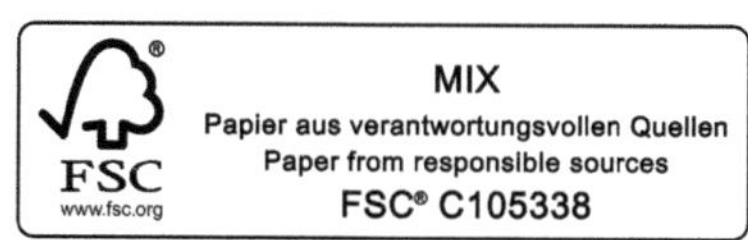

Printed by Books on Demand GmbH, Norderstedt / Germany